HEALING
THE WHOLE PERSON

DR HIRA SINGH

Published in the United States by Hill of Content Publishing

Published in the United Kingdom by Hill of Content Publishing

Published in Australia by Hill of Content Publishing

Published in India by Hill of Content Publishing

Distributed by Etoile International Group. Hong Kong.

hillofcontentpublishing.com

PO Box 24 East Melbourne 8002 Victoria Australia

Cover design: Yasmine Davidson * *Interior design:* Will Gerard

National Library of Australia Cataloguing-in-Publication data:

Singh, Hira,
Healing the Whole Person

Includes index: ISBN: 978-0-6483443-5-3

*This book is dedicated to all those who seek to
understand Healing*

———

*May all sentient beings everywhere be free of Suffering, and the
roots of their Suffering.*

*May all sentient beings everywhere find Joy and Contentment
within themselves.*

May I be free of my Suffering, and the roots of my Suffering.

May I find Joy and Contentment within myself.

"I am honoured and grateful to have met Dr Singh over 30 years ago. For decades he has dedicated himself to teaching doctors, medical students, and the community on the value of holistic health care in the most ethical way. He is a great teacher. This book is a culmination of Dr Singh's lifetime work, knowledge, and wisdom."

Associate Professor Vicki Kotsirilos
AM MBBS FACNEM FASLM
Awarded Hon. Fellow RACGP
Founding President The Australasian
Integrative Medicine Association

PREFACE

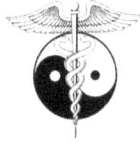

This logo reflects the integrated use of complementary insights and techniques developed from both Eastern and Western traditions of healing. In the background is the T'ai-chi T'u, which means 'Diagram of the Supreme Ultimate', or more popularly known as Yin-Yang.

In the oriental world-view, the circle represents the whole, which is made up of two inter-penetrating and opposing forces (darkness and light), which naturally balance and complement each other.

Superimposed on this is the Staff of Hermes, the symbol of Hippocratic medicine, representing the traditional roots of modern medicine. In even more ancient symbolism the entwined serpents represent the twin nadis, or channels along which the Vital Energy rises, passing through the chakras, or centres of consciousness, which correspond to the plexuses of the Autonomic Nervous system; the centre staff representing the spinal cord.

FOREWORD

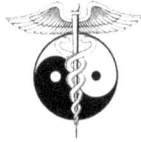

In *Healing the Whole Person* Dr Hira Singh brings together his wealth of experience over decades working as an Integrative Medicine (IM) doctor in general practice. He is a pioneer of integrative medicine in Australia. Dr Singh has experience in most of the modalities that are part of the integrative approach, which very few clinicians have. These include Acupuncture, Biofeedback, Spinal Manipulation, Nutritional Medicine, Stress Management (Meditation) and Counselling. He has been active in the education of clinicians and the public and was a founding board member of the Australasian Integrative Medicine Association.

Integrative medicine combines mainstream medicine with evidence-based complementary medicine to achieve optimal outcomes in health improvement, prevention and treatment of illness. A key part of IM has to do with *why* a person has developed their illness, hence providing the best opportunity for the patient's healing. It is becoming clear that the most important factors leading to the development of illness relate to behavioural issues.

When we look at health from a 'whole person' perspective, many human factors contribute to our health and wellbeing, from the physical to mind-body influences. This book explores a range of human factors such as loneliness, happiness, grief, stress, forgiveness, anger, fear etc., and offers practical advice on how to resolve these issues. It offers us simple, effective ways we can all follow to improve our lifestyle for health optimisation and personal growth. It provides a road map for the 'whole person' approach, which offers the best that all medicine has to offer. It would also be a very useful educational resource for any clinician who is keen on expanding their toolbox when treating patients.

I would highly recommend this book for anyone looking to improve their health and wellbeing, at all stages of life.

Professor Avni Sali AM MBBS PhD FRACS FACS FACNEM
Founder & Director – National Institute of Integrative Medicine

CONTENTS

INTRODUCTION

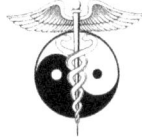

I have written this book as a guide for self-care in response to requests from my patients. It is the outline on which I have based my approach to consulting during the forty-five years of my work in Australian General Practice.

With increasingly easy access to health information on the internet, more patients are expecting their doctor to engage with them on their health journey. They request explanations, question their prescriptions, and are not content to be passive recipients of a paternalistic medical culture. The doctor-God image just doesn't cut it any more.

The practitioner and the patient must share responsibility for the healing process. Releasing the doctor from the 'rescuer' role prevents practitioner burnout, while releasing the patient from the 'victim' role encourages a healthier dynamic that acknowledges the role of personal attitudes and lifestyle in the process of healing.

This book reflects my own understanding of health and illness, which emphasises the 'Whole Person' approach. By this I mean looking beyond the physical signs and symptoms of disease to find their wider context in the mental, emotional and spiritual life of the patient, and formulating a plan of management, which can result in not merely the resolution of the patient's physical distress but also lead to self-empowering personal growth.

This goes beyond the usual biomedical or conventional model, which constrains many time-poor practitioners. By going beyond mere symptom resolution to explore the context of the illness in the patient's life, this whole-person approach offers a more satisfying way of helping patients achieve optimal health outcomes.

In the following chapters this approach will become clearer as I discuss in more detail the major influences on health and make suggestions for improving individual self-care. However, this is not an academic text, nor is it meant to replace professional medical advice.

The 'Whole Person' is a multi-dimensional being with physical, emotional, mental, and spiritual aspects functioning in an environment which impacts on their health. Being linear, our language forces us to discuss these aspects in separate chapters. In so doing, we risk the loss of the integrated, interrelated dynamic, which is the whole person.

To embed this understanding as a foundation of my practice I have included in Chapter Two a brief overview, highlighting the historical and philosophical background supporting my whole-person position. The reader may wish to skip this chapter and just read the relevant sections on the various aspects of the whole person, but I would recommend reading Chapter Two beforehand, to be informed of the wider context in which the chapters that follow are anchored.

I have also included some specific case studies to illustrate how the whole-person approach has led to significantly improved health outcomes for my patients.

Hira Singh

1

WHAT IS HEALTH?

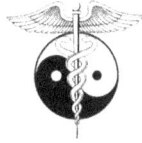

Healing is transformation, an essential process for growth, a movement from dis-ease to a new dynamic balance, which allows for a fuller expression of life in the individual.

The World Health Organisation's definition of Health is:

A state of complete physical, mental and social wellbeing, and not merely the absence of disease and infirmity.

The Well-being Institute at the University of Cambridge defines wellbeing as:

...a positive and sustainable characteristic which enables individuals and organisations to thrive and flourish.

These definitions are aligned with the whole-person approach, which I have used in my own practice.

To me health is a dynamic state of wellness in which there is homeostasis (balance) while maintaining equilibrium with the environment, which then allows for optimal functioning. This means we must acknowledge the influences of mental/emotional states on the physical body. Scientific studies in the field of psycho-neuro-immunology have amply researched and documented these interrelationships.

This paradigm shift from the conventional biomedical to the bio-psycho-social model was at first called 'Holistic/ Wholistic Medicine'. Today it is termed 'Integrative Medicine'. 'Lifestyle Medicine' is another term that encompasses similar thinking. Some refer to it as 'Network Medicine' or 'Functional Medicine'.

In his *Wellness Workbook* (1981), Dr John Travis illustrated this understanding of health as a continuum, expressed in the following chart.

Illness progresses to the left of the continuum on the chart on the next page, with the appearance of subjective signs and symptoms. If these are missed or ignored and left untreated, then a functional disturbance will lead to structural changes indicating physical illness. Unsuccessful treatment at this stage will lead to disability and premature death.

ILLNESS / WELLNESS CONTINUUM

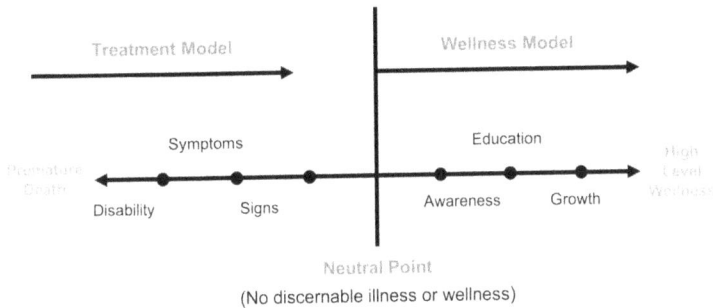

Treatment Model

Wellness Model

Symptoms

Education

Premature Death

Disability

Signs

Awareness

Growth

High Level Wellness

Neutral Point

(No discernable illness or wellness)

The movement to Wellness progresses to the right of the neutral point on the continuum, with a patient's developing awareness of changes in the functioning of their own system. Patients educated to develop preventive self-care habits and to participate in screening programs for at-risk diseases, and encouraged to develop a sense of personal responsibility, can be guided through their growth into high-level wellness; 'to thrive and flourish' as The Wellbeing Institute puts it.

The Wellness model aims to optimise high-level functioning. In this state the body-mind is functioning with such a clarity of purpose that it allows the life force its natural creative expression, unobstructed and undistorted. We associate this state of wellness with joy, creativity and a sense of fulfilment and contentment. This is what the Wholistic/Integrative medical model aims to do.

The treatment model works on the left of the neutral point on the chart. Its job is done when symptoms/signs of disease are eliminated, and basic functionality is restored. This is mainly what the 'Allopathic' or biomedical model (also known as 'conventional' or 'mainstream' medicine), usually encompasses.

What Is Healing?

There is healing when there is true attunement with the life process. There is healing when the illusion of our being a separate self, vulnerable and self-centred is replaced by surrender to, communion with, and identification with the limitless whole of which everyone and everything is part.

Frances Horn PhD, psychotherapist.

Healing is transformation, an essential process for growth, a movement from dis-ease to a new dynamic balance which allows for a fuller expression of life in the individual. It involves change, which in turn means letting go of patterns of conditioning that have become inappropriate, restrictive and inhibitive to the flow of life energy.

True healing always involves a shift in consciousness. By overcoming the resistance to change, the individual is freed from the constrictive experience of dis-ease to embrace a new expanded sense of self.

The call of illness is a challenge, which can only be met by trusting in an innate intelligence, ever-present in every individual, yet hidden until called upon. It involves the surrender of the ego-self. The more fully we surrender this, the deeper will be our healing.

The healer is a catalyst helping to bring about this transformation. He/she could be a sympathetic friend, an empathic counsellor, a trusted teacher, or a health practitioner. I have witnessed significant resolution of chronic and debilitating health conditions brought about by creating a safe space and guiding the patient to discover meaning in suffering; by non-judgemental support; and by encouraging a hopeful attitude.

The medical consultation is a unique opportunity to create such a change. In the interaction of a consultation there is reciprocal movement and exchange of energy between practitioner and patient, but judgement stops this interaction. Whereas an open and respectful acceptance of the patient's experience as valid allows movement into new possibilities. In this safe space imbued with an atmosphere of trust, infused with hope, love, and empathy, the alchemy of healing may reveal itself as a conscious transformative experience.

2

MEDICINE THROUGH HISTORY

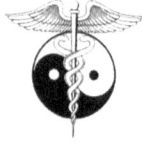

The great error of the day is that physicians separate the soul from the body.

- PLATO

In prehistoric times the medicine-man was a magician-physician. He interpreted undesirable changes in nature as the result of malign forces and used charms and incantations, herbs and plants to effect cures.

Evidence of this can be found in studies of our own Australian Aboriginal people, who can trace their ancestry in Australia to more than 60,000 years ago.

From around 4000 BCE we have records from the civilisations which established themselves around the Tigris and Euphrates Rivers – the cultures of Mesopotamia, Sumeria, Babylon and Assyria. Their medical practice was directly linked to prehistoric magic and empirical herbal lore, but it shifted into the hands of priests and lay physicians. It was based on the observation of natural phenomena, astrology and cycles in nature. The interaction between the microcosm (man) and the macrocosm (Universe) was the underlying philosophy used to explain the experience of illness.

The history of western civilisation is rooted in ancient Greece. The culture of Greece's 'Milesian' school of thought, around 600 BCE, did not distinguish among science, philosophy, and religion. The term 'physics' is coined from the Greek word *physis*, which means the endeavour of seeing the essential nature of all things. This definition has a strongly mystical flavour and aptly describes the spiritual search embarked upon by the early mystics.

These early Greeks were called 'Hylozoists', which meant they were 'those who think matter is alive', because they saw no distinction between animate and inanimate, spirit and matter, but saw each characteristic as interdiffused with the other. Heraclitus, a Greek philosopher of the sixth century BCE, taught that all changes in the world arise from the dynamic and cyclic interplay of opposites, and he saw any pair of opposites as a 'Unity'. He called this unity 'the Logos'. This view is virtually identical with the eastern concept of 'Yin-Yang' – the mutual interdependence and balance of all phenomena. Heraclitus is best remembered for his famous aphorism: *Panta rhei* – 'Everything flows'.

It was another Greek, Pythagoras, together with his contemporary Alcmaeon of Croton (around 500 BCE), who laid the foundation of what later became known as 'Hippocratic medicine'. He gave us the concept of 'isonomia'. According to this concept 'health' is a state of perfect harmony, 'disease' is an expression of disturbance of this harmony, and 'cure' is a return from the disturbed to the harmonious state. It sounds so simple and obvious yet, apart from the period of Hippocratic medicine, this concept of health as a state of perfect harmony was abandoned by subsequent models of healthcare. Today our practice is the poorer for its neglect of this earlier understanding.

Hippocrates, who is often hailed as 'the father of modern medicine', lived on the Greek island of Kos from 460 to about 370 BCE. He established the practice of medicine as both a science and an art, freeing it from the domination of priests and temples. He based his practice on strict observation of the patient and noted how the seasons, climate, environment, diet and lifestyle affected the physical and psychic life of the individual. His wholistic outlook is summarised in his statement that it is more important for the physician to know what kind of person has a disease, rather than to know what kind of disease a person has.

His invaluable contribution to medicine is that he established the fact that disease is a natural process; that symptoms are the reactions of the body to the disease, and that the physician's chief role is to support the natural forces of the body in their move towards recovery. One of Hippocrates' most famous aphorisms is: 'First do no harm'.

The Dawn of Duality

Divergence from the Heraclitean 'Unity' view discussed above began with the 'Eleatic' school of thought in the fifth century BCE, which assumed a divine principle standing above all gods and humans and separate from observed nature.

This eventually led to the concept of the atom as the smallest and indivisible unit of matter. The 'Atomists' believed that matter and spirit were two different things and that material inert particles, atoms, were somehow moving in the void, directed by external and eternal forces assumed to be of spiritual origin. Thus was born the concept of the duality of mind and matter, the separation between body and soul. This disintegrated view of humankind led the renowned Greek philosopher Plato (late fifth century BCE) to say:

> *The great error of the day is that physicians separate the soul from the body.*

Today, more than 2,500 years later, our practice of medicine continues to perpetuate this 'great error'. Slowly, in the following few centuries, the Hippocratic idea of medicine lost ground and its practical concepts crystallised into the rigidity and dogma of formulae. Theoretical interpretation rather than practical observation now formed the basis of medicine. From this point on, western thought was preoccupied with this division between matter and spirit. Philosophers turned their attention to the spiritual world, while Aristotelian deductive logic and inductive analysis (named for its originator, the fourth-century BCE Greek philosopher Aristotle), dominated the western view of the universe for the next 2,000 years; supported by the Christian church throughout the Middle Ages. We will skip these dark ages when purging and bloodletting dominated the practice of medicine to pick up our thread in the period of the Renaissance, around the sixteenth century CE, when science started to establish itself as an experimental model of nature.

Two important personalities were involved in the paradigm that dominated western thinking from the mid-seventeenth to the end of the nineteenth century CE. The first is René Descartes – the seventeenth-century French philosopher (also a mathematician and physiologist), who divided nature into two separate and independent parts: in Latin, *Res cogitans* (the mind) and *Res extensa* (matter). His famous statement: *Cogito ergo sum* – 'I think, therefore I am', has led western humankind to equate the individual's existence with his/her mind, instead of the whole organism including the body. Consequently, we now see ourselves as isolated egos existing inside our separate bodies This inner fragmentation of humankind mirrors Descartes' (Cartesian) view of the outside world, which he saw as a multitude of separate objects and events to be manipulated for our individual good.

The second personality was the eighteenth-century English physicist Isaac Newton, who based his theories of classical physics on a mechanistic world view wherein life and the universe constituted a great cosmic machine which could be understood by breaking it down into its component parts. Science thus saw the human body too as a machine which could be understood by dissecting it into its basic building-block parts.

'Isonomia': 'Health' is a state of perfect harmony, 'disease' is an expression of disturbance of this harmony, and 'cure' is a return from the disturbed to the harmonious state.

— *PYTHAGORAS AND ALCMAEON OF CROTON*

From these Cartesian and Newtonian world views developed the present-day biomedical model and with it the advent of specialist physicians and surgeons who study the structure and function of the different parts of the body exclusively and independently as if they were unconnected. Great advances in technology and science allow doctors today to intervene ever more aggressively to rectify disorders at the physical level, replace diseased organs through surgery, and prolong patients' lives with potent chemicals. We now have 'super specialists' who make a good living by dealing exclusively with only one small part of the body.

In his book *The Turning Point,* Fritjof Capra writes:

The mechanistic view of the human organism has encouraged an engineering approach to health in which illness is reduced to mechanical trouble and medical therapy to technical manipulation. An important aspect of this view...is the belief that the cure of illness requires some outside intervention by the physician. Modern medicine often loses sight of the patient as a human being. In fact, the question "What is health?" is generally not even addressed in medical schools, nor is there any discussion of healthy attitudes and lifestyles. These are considered philosophical issues that belong to the spiritual realm, outside the domain of Medicine.

Modern Physics Harks Back to Connection

Ironically, while modern medicine was busy shackling itself to this mechanistic model to gain credibility and respectability as a scientific discipline, modern physics was starting to explore the relationship between consciousness and matter.

By the end of the nineteenth century, Quantum Theory and Einstein's Theory of Relativity were showing that matter and energy were two interchangeable forms of the one phenomenon. This insight describes the universe as *undivided wholeness in flowing movement,* in the words of twentieth-century American-Brazilian-English physicist David Bohm. In this flow, mind and matter are not separate substances. Rather, they are different aspects of one whole and unbroken movement. This revelation reminds us of Heraclitus: 'Everything flows'.

A century later we still find it difficult to recognise these insights of quantum physics; we continue to be dominated by the Cartesian-Newtonian model of fragmentation among body, mind, and spirit. Yet, as we have seen from this historical review, a wholistic, organic, interrelated four-dimensional understanding of the universe and ourselves is not new. The early Greeks knew this, and mystics throughout the centuries have described reality through similar ideas.

It has taken physics to bring us full circle to acknowledge the connectedness of all phenomena, including humankind, within a multidimensional organism. All things, and we too, are an integral part of this underlying whole.

3

WHOLE-PERSON CARE

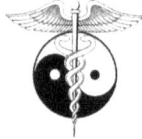

Each person is unique and their health management should be individualised. What may work for one, may not work for another.

The whole person-focused approach to healthcare is grounded in the wholistic understanding and recognition of the biological, psychological, and social influences that affect the individual's wellbeing.

This means the health practitioner must engage with the patient as a whole person so that the complaint they are presenting can be considered in the context of their life situation. This approach goes beyond the doctor's immediate concern to relieve distress and involves an exploration of the patient's beliefs, lifestyle, and behaviour. In this sense, each person is unique and their health management should be individualised. What may work for one, may not work for another.

The doctor and the patient share responsibility for the healing process. Releasing the doctor from the 'rescuer' role prevents practitioner burnout, while releasing the patient from the 'victim' role encourages a healthier dynamic that acknowledges the active role of personal attitudes and lifestyle on the process of healing.

Usually, the illness experience is seen as a crisis requiring intervention. This is true for medical emergencies, to which our advances in technology provide an excellent response. However, for many non-acute presentations seen at the primary care level, we could serve the patient better by guiding them to examine where changes in their attitude and lifestyle could restore balance. Clarifying the context in which the illness appears can help the patient to find meaning in the suffering and see it as a creative opportunity. Assuming personal responsibility, developing insight, and then making fundamental changes may not only resolve the illness but result in the patient's growth into wellness.

Going beyond the diagnosis and treatment stages of intervention involves the doctor or practitioner taking on the role of educator and health coach. Adopting preventive health habits empowers the patient to become an active participant in their own healing journey rather than a passive and unquestioning recipient of suppressive therapies. In helping patients with chronic illnesses for which no quick resolution is expected, the doctor becomes a mentor, committed to staying the course by the patient's side, supporting, and encouraging them with small changes to better manage the situation.

Western medicine is not the only available
path to better healthcare.

There are other models of understanding illness and health. Complementary care involving other therapies has been shown to have beneficial effects: Yoga, Tai Chi, Qi Gong, Pilates, meditation, hypnotherapy, acupuncture, physiotherapy, naturopathy and even music and humour therapy, among others, can all contribute to a wellness program.

General dissatisfaction with conventional care drives the demand for such alternative therapies. No one system can claim exclusive rights to understanding the entire ambit of health and illness. A respectful attitude to so-called 'unconventional' therapies brings a better understanding of their role. If the practitioner acknowledges the limitations of each of these therapies, they can be deployed to work together in the interest of the patient. As important as healing skills are in themselves, it is the practitioner's attitude when using these skills that is critical to delivering the desired outcome.

The practitioner working with the 'whole person' model aims to inform, educate, and encourage the patient about healthy lifestyle behaviours, and seeks to create a safe atmosphere for doctor-patient interaction so that healing can take place.

There is evidence that chronic diseases like diabetes, obesity, heart disease, neuro-degenerative diseases and some cancers are linked to unhealthy lifestyle behaviours. The American College of Lifestyle Medicine, founded in 2021, estimates that 60% of American adults have at least one chronic disease and 40% have two chronic diseases. The US$4.1 trillion spent annually to support the current healthcare model in the United States is now recognised as unsustainable. A similar situation exists in most countries, including Australia, where the 'drug-and-disease' paradigm dominates the medical and research professions.

Instead, we could bring about improved outcomes in health and manage many conditions, just by using primary means such as lifestyle behaviour changes in nutrition, physical activity, sleep, stress management, social connections and the abuse of risky substances. This way, we could keep medications and many surgical or other procedures in reserve as adjunct treatments only. This would address rising healthcare costs, as well as lead to improved practitioner and patient satisfaction.

The University of South Carolina's School of Medicine Greenville has taken the initiative by introducing Lifestyle Medicine modules into all four years of its curriculum. My hope is that our medical schools in Australia could at least follow in this same direction, as this required change in emphasis is best started at the student level.

This wholistic model does not deny the great achievements of medical technology that serve us so well in medical emergencies, trauma management and surgery, but it does go further beyond the limited perspectives of such technology. This is the model that restores the missing dimension in contemporary medical practice – to stop seeing the human individual as a separate, fragmented ego-self, but rather as a whole person connected with life, as 'an undivided wholeness in flowing movement.' (David Bohm).

Case Study 1: A 'Burnt-out' Professional

John, who was a 48-year-old solicitor and a senior partner in a successful practice, reported to me about his recently increasing irritability, disturbed sleep, fatigue, reduced libido and feeling 'burnt-out'.

He had been busy working long hours on a difficult case, which was being delayed through no fault of his. This left him feeling frustrated and helpless.

I first suggested some simple changes to his diet with more regular meals and reducing alcohol and caffeine. He had started a walking schedule three times a week and I encouraged him to aim for a half-hour brisk walk five times a week. I also taught him abdominal breathing and how to invoke the relaxation response. (See next page and Chapter 4 for these strategies). He found that remembering to pause and briefly shift to deep breathing many times in the day made him less tired. He used coloured dot stickers on his bathroom mirror, phone, fridge, and computer screen as reminder cues to bring his awareness into the present moment. He also set aside fifteen minutes in the morning to sit quietly and practise mindfulness meditation, which he found useful in setting a more measured tone for the rest of his workday.

Subsequent counselling sessions focused on examining his perfectionist tendencies, readjusting personal standards, releasing self-critical thoughts, and repeating affirmations. Four weeks later John reported feeling more in charge of his life, experiencing deeply restful states with his practice of relaxation, and was planning a long-overdue holiday with his family.

John's case reminded me of how easily work demands can result in self-neglect and push people to slip into maladaptive behaviour. Many middle-aged men in business or the professions who hold leadership or executive positions tend to deny the stress they feel and choose to 'plough on' rather than be seen as 'weak' if they seek help. Sometimes it takes the harsh message of a health crisis to jolt them into better self-care.

Relaxation Exercise

Place yourself in a comfortable position. Let your mind drift through your body and check that everywhere is loose, relaxed, and unrestricted by clothing or an uncomfortable position. Make whatever minor adjustments you might need to make yourself comfortable. Take a couple of long, slow, deep breaths, in and out, as you let your eyes close.

Let your attention drift to the very top of your head, to your scalp and forehead, smoothing out all the muscles in your scalp and your forehead. Just let them go, relax them.

Continue to let this relaxation flow over your cheeks, lips, and chin. Relax your whole face. Pay special attention to your jaw, just letting the muscles go.

Let go of your tongue, your throat, and your vocal cords, letting your vocal cords become quiet.

Let the relaxation continue to flow down the back of your head, letting go of the muscles in your neck and shoulders. Smooth out those tiny knots in your muscles. Untie them and let them lie limp.

Continue to relax your shoulders and let that warmth spread down your upper arms, relaxing all the muscles of your upper arm down to your elbows, your forearms. Let go of the muscles around your wrists and hands, your fingertips. Let them be comfortable and heavy. As you let go of the tension, the blood flows more easily into the fingertips.

Smooth out all the muscles along your shoulders and upper back. Continue to relax all the way down into your lower back along your spine. Smooth out all the muscles in your waist and buttocks. Let that relaxation come around the sides of your body, letting go of the muscles around your rib cage. With every breath, allow your chest to become more and more relaxed...just observe it.

Let go of all the muscles around your hips, waist and pelvis.

This relaxation flows down to your thighs, knees, shins, calves, letting your legs become heavy, comfortable and relaxed. Let go of your ankles, heels, feet, even the soles of your feet and toes. As your legs become relaxed, blood flows more easily to the toes and warms your feet.

Your whole body feels relaxed, peaceful and calm...

The Relaxation Response

Arrange not to be disturbed.

Sit comfortably, hands in your lap, legs uncrossed, and gently close your eyes.

Take a couple of deep breaths. Relax your body beginning with the muscles in your head and face, repeating through your body down to your toes. Breathe in through your nose. As you exhale, say the word 'ONE' silently to yourself, and continue saying it each time you breathe out.

Continue to relax and become calm. If you notice tensions in your muscles, relax them. If thoughts come into your mind or noises distract you, just return to repeating 'ONE'. Let the thoughts go. Don't get caught up in them. Continue for ten to twenty minutes.

When you finish, open your eyes slowly. Sit for a moment, stretch, and enjoy the relaxation.

4

PHYSICAL

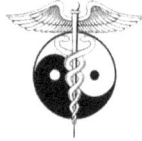

Physical activity in the form of regular exercise benefits not only the body but also contributes to mental and emotional wellbeing.

The physical body is usually the first place where we register distress, either as pain or impaired function. It is also the dominant, for some the exclusive, reality that we identify with as our individual self. Yet the body is not merely a solid structure of organs, bones and muscles encased in a skin as it appears to us. It is a dynamic self-regulating system of energy in constant exchange with its environment. Every atom in the body is replaced every two years, a new liver is formed every six weeks, and a new stomach lining every four weeks. Food, water, and oxygen are the three essential sources of nourishment that the body needs for its healthy growth and function.

But a healthy body also requires movement. Physical activity in the form of regular exercise benefits not only the body, but also contributes to mental and emotional wellbeing. To maintain healthy biorhythms, we need to balance our activity with rest periods and sleep.

Even small changes in all the areas described below can result in a significant initial improvement in physical wellbeing. This improvement can act as motivation to encourage us toward more lifestyle changes once the immediate crisis has been managed. After that, we can consider further exploration of the underlying belief system related to the illness.

Nutrition

We have created a complex relationship with food in our modern world.

Our behaviour around food, beyond fulfilling energy requirements, may reflect an unrecognised or unmet need in other areas of our lives. An imbalance in body-image issues or significant family relationships often underlies the dysfunctional eating patterns observed in eating disorders such as anorexia and bulimia.

Eating on the run, skipping meals, or reaching for convenient pre-packed food when we are busy, are all habits that reflect our lack of attentiveness to our bodies' fundamental need for good food. To honour this need we must make time, sit down with family or friends for a meal where possible, enjoy the aroma and presentation, savour the taste, and give thanks for the sustenance the food provides. We can achieve this by 'becoming present' during the eating experience. Chewing our food before we too hastily swallow it is the important first step in digestion. Remember, there are no teeth inside the stomach!

The food that we eat is only as good as the soil, air, and water in which it has been grown.

Deforestation, excessive cropping, and grazing have all contributed to depletion of the topsoil in Australia and New Zealand, resulting in low levels of selenium and zinc, among other trace minerals. The chemical fertilisers that are then added to compensate for such mineral losses and to enrich the soil affect the natural resistance of plants and grains to pests. Pesticides are then sprayed to protect against crop losses. The chemical burden is increased when unripe fruits are picked, then needing to be irradiated and sometimes waxed to appeal to the supermarket shopper. Yet another layer of chemicals comes with the food additives, added to processed and packaged foods to stabilise and preserve them. These may include flavourings, colourings, and preservatives. For some sensitive individuals, even the so-called 'safe' regulated levels of chemical exposure may provoke food intolerances and allergies. It is good practice to wash and peel fruits and vegetables before cooking.

At the time of writing there are at least twelve chemicals (pesticides and herbicides), which are still being used in Australia but which have been banned overseas for their adverse health effects. Among these are Paraquat (linked to Parkinson's disease), Atrazine (impacting human reproduction and coral reef ecosystems), Chlorpyrifos (causing brain damage in children), and Neonicotinoids (toxic to honey bees, hence affecting the pollination of plants and crops).

It should come as no surprise that the nutritional value of our food has declined as compared with pre-industrial times, given the scale and practice of modern farming and animal husbandry. A movement to improve the quality of our food has begun, with more people now favouring and seeking out organically grown produce. The food industry is also taking note of this trend.

Most people are familiar with the Five Food Groups:

1. Bread and cereals
2. Fruits and vegetables
3. Fish, eggs, meat, and nuts
4. Milk, cheese and yoghurt
5. Butter and margarine

The first two groups should account for 75% of the food we eat, yet the typical Australian diet has only 30% from these groups, together with 45% from fats and 25% from sugars.

Various studies have highlighted the relationship between such dietary patterns and the increasing incidence of obesity, strokes, heart disease, cancers, gut disorders and allergies. All degenerative diseases commonly progress from inflammation through oxidative and metabolic stress linked with a pituitary-adrenal imbalance that has been impacted by the gut microbiome. Chemical compounds as well as biological agents (viruses, bacteria, fungi), trigger the first phase of inflammation in the gut. This results in damage to the protective and absorptive lining of the gut, allowing peptides (incompletely broken down amino-acid chains), to enter the circulatory system. These in turn provoke a reaction from the immune system, which recognises them as 'foreign' (antigens), and sets out to neutralise them by creating antibodies (antigen-'fighter proteins'). The resulting biological storm from antigen-antibody conflict further stresses the cell's ability to maintain its balance. Degeneration increases rapidly from here.

Social media, with the aid of celebrities and influencers, promote a plethora of diets which promise to make you younger/healthier/stronger/slimmer. These diets are often restrictive in their choice of foods, potentially unhealthy over the long term, and usually unsustainable as a long-term life choice.

The Low Stress Diet is a guide to healthy eating suitable for all ages. It reduces or avoids exposure to common reactive foods, while providing alternatives to retain a good balance of essential nutrients.

LOW STRESS DIET

CATEGORY	FOOD RECOMMENDED	FOOD TO AVOID
MEATS	FISH, CHICKEN, LAMB, BEEF, PORK	PROCESSES MEATS, POLONY, SALAMI, SAUSAGE, SHELLFISH
DAIRY PRODUCTS	PLAIN YOGURT (LIVE CULTURE BUTTERMILK, WHEY)	MILK, CHEESE & ALL PRODUCTS CONTAINING THEM
OTHER PROTEINS	EGGS	
GRAINS	RYE GRAINS & FLOUR (RYVITA, WUPPER, OTHER RYE BREADS), MILLET BUCKWHEAT, OATS, BROWN RICE	WHEAT & ALL WHEAT PRODUCTS (BRAN, WHEATGERM, MALT)
NUTS	ALMONDS	PEANUTS, COCONUT
SEEDS	ALL SEEDS (SESAME, SUNFLOWER, PEPITAS, LINSEED)	NONE
VEGETABLES	ALL VEGETABLES (RAW, STEAMED, SAUTEED OR BAKED)	CANNED OR FROZEN VEGES, MUSHROOMS, OLIVES
LEGUMES	BEANS, CHICKPEAS, LENTILS, SOYABEANS	
SPROUTS	ALL SPROUTS	NONE
FRUIT	ALL FRESH FRUITS	CANNED, DRIED OR FROZEN VEGES, MUSHROOMS, OLIVES
SWEETS	HONEY, CAROB	ALL SUGARS, CHOCOLATE, SYRUPS, & ALL PRODUCTS CONTAINING THEM
SEASONINGS	ALL HERBS	ALL SPICES, BLACK & WHITE PEPPER
CONDIMENTS	OLIVE OIL, SUGARLESS SAUCES	VINEGAR, SOY SAUCE, MISO, MUSTARD, PICKLES, MAYONNAISE, & ALL SAUCES CONTAINING THEM
SPREADS	TAHINI, RAW HONEY HOME MADE SPREADS, SUGAR FREE JAMS	VEGEMITE, MARMITE, PROMITE, PEANUT BUTTER, SWEETENED JAMS
OILS	COLD PRESSED VEGETABLE & SEED OILS, CANOLA	NUT OILS, POLYUNSATURATED OILS
BEVERAGES	HERB TEAS, PURE FRESH JUICES, COFFEE SUBSTITUTES E.G. CARO, DECAF TEA & COFFEE	ALL ALCOHOL, COFFEE, TEA, CANNED JUICES, CARBONATED SOFT DRINKS CONTAINING ADDED SUGAR PRESERVATIVES & COLOUR
YEAST	NONE	ALL PRODUCTS CONTAINING BREWERS YEAST, TORULA YEAST, BAKERS YEAST INCLUDING SOME VITAMIN SUPPLEMENTS
WATER	6-8 GLASSES PER DAY	

Another consideration is the acid-alkaline balance in the body. For the best metabolism, the pH of the body is maintained between 7.35 and 7.45, a slightly alkaline state, with the ideal around 7.4. This balancing regulation is the combined work of the lungs (oxygen-carbon dioxide exchange), and the kidneys (electrolyte balance). This is the reason correct breathing and adequate hydration are so important. This vital balance is best served by eating a diet which has 70% to 80% alkaline-forming foods.

Whole foods should be the first choice for good nutrition, while vitamin supplements should be reserved for short-term nutrition replacement when needed.

Acid and Alkaline Foods

The body seems to work best on a diet high in alkaline-forming foods - those foods which give alkaline elements when broken down by the digestion. A diet which contains 70% - 80% alkaline-forming foods is ideal for healthful living.

Fruits
Acid
cranberries
pomegranates
strawberries
sour fruits

Alkaline
apples
bananas
citrus fruits
dates
grapes
cherries
peaches
pears
plums
papaya
mangoes
pineapple
raspberries
blackberries
huckleberries
elderberries
boysenberries
persimmons
apricots
olives
coconut
figs
raisins
melons

Vegetables
All vegetables are alkaline (includes starchy vegetables like potatoes, squash and parsnips.)

Grains
Acid
Brown Rice
Barley
Wheat
Oats
Rye
Breads

Alkaline
Millet
Buckwheat
Corn
Sprouted grains

Meats and Diary Products
Acid
All meats
Fish
Fowl
Eggs
Cheese
Milk
Yogurt
Butter

Alkaline
Non-fat milk

Nuts
Acid
Cashews
Walnuts
Filberts
Peanuts
Pecans
Macadamia nuts

Alkaline
Almonds
Brazil nuts

Seeds
Acid
Pumpkin
Sesame
Sunflower
Chia
Flax

Alkaline
All sprouted seeds

Beans and Peas
Acid
Lentils
Navy
Aduki
Kidney

Alkaline
Soybeans
Limas
Sprouted beans

Sugars
Acid
Brown sugar
White sugar
Milk sugar
Cane syrup
Malt syrup
Maple syrup
Molasses

Alkaline
Honey

Oils
Acid
Nut oils
Butter
Cream

Alkaline
Olive Oil
Soy
Sesame
Sunflower
Corn
Safflower
Cottonseed
Margarine

The gut microbiome has attracted much attention in recent years. Research in this field, though still in its early stage, has revealed direct interactions between the gut flora (the microorganisms that live in our intestines) and multiple organ systems. The impact of the gut microbiome on a diverse range of disorders includes even mental and emotional states through its biological dysregulation of key neuropeptides and neurotransmitters essential for stable brain function. Not only can a poor diet create imbalance in the gut microbiome, but repeated doses of antibiotics may also harm it, along with some oral chemotherapy drugs that target rapidly multiplying cells. Our best and recommended protection against such side-effects is to use prebiotics (plant-fibre foods like broccoli, cauliflower, etc.), that feed 'good' bacteria in the gut, and probiotics such as plain yoghurt that already host living 'good' bacteria.

Less well studied at this stage are the roles that the skin surface microbiome and the uro-genital tract microbiome play in conditions which affect the skin and the urinary system respectively.

Food Intolerance

It is important to distinguish between allergy and intolerance.

True food allergy is indicated by the presence in the body of an antibody (usually immunoglobulin E). The body creates such an antibody when it detects a 'foreign substance' or antigen (a food protein/peptide), which has been absorbed in the small intestine. The antibody is the body's response to this antigen's 'invasion'. The resulting antigen-antibody complex then reacts at the surface of the 'mast cell' (white blood cells most commonly found on the skin and intestinal tract), and this reaction releases chemicals like histamine, which are responsible for the allergic reaction. The reaction could be an immediate hypersensitivity reaction, or it could be delayed by days, as in the case of migraines. Nut allergy in children is an example of a true food allergy.

Intolerance on the other hand is often dosage - or quantity - related: it usually involves multiple food substances that either singulary or in combination accumulate to exceed a threshold preferred by the body.

Toxic reactions can arise from naturally occurring chemicals in some foods: for example, alkaloids in potatoes; salicylates in fruits and vegetables; theobromine in chocolates; caffeine in tea and coffee; amines (histamine, tyramine, serotonin, phenylalanine) found in cheese, sausages and fermented foods; and oxalic acid in rhubarb and spinach. 'Mast Cell Activation Syndrome' is a relatively new term covering a range of chronic symptoms brought about by these food chemicals. Food additives like preservatives, antioxidants, artificial colouring agents, artificial sweeteners and flavours can also cause reactions in sensitive individuals. Additionally, the hyperactivity that we see in children who exhibit disruptive behaviour, short attention spans, poor sleeping patterns and poor muscle coordination also stems from such food additives.

'Chinese restaurant syndrome' is well recognised now as being caused by a reaction to monosodium glutamate (MSG) seasoning used in some Chinese meals, producing symptoms such as chest pain, burning skin, headaches, palpitations, sweating, and nausea, and even provoking asthma attacks in known asthmatics. This reaction is usually worse in people with low vitamin B6 levels.

Eliminating certain preservatives and additives from the diet (such as tartrazine, sodium benzoate, brewer's yeast, sodium salicylate and sodium metabisulphite) can relieve certain skin disorders like chronic urticaria (itchy rash, hives etc.).

For sensitive individuals with symptoms suggestive of food intolerance, an elimination diet is usually prescribed and is worth trialling This entails a process where the doctor and patient together chart the patient's reactions/non-reactions to specific foods by avoiding them for set periods of time, to identify which food may be responsible for the allergic reaction. This is followed by slowly reintroducing the identified offending foods once every three to four days on a rotation basis to further check on any possible reaction. Restoring the biodiversity of the gut microbiome in this way also helps to reduce the reactivity of the system. The elimination diet is best supervised by a health practitioner trained in nutrition.

Supplements

Micronutrient supplementation is a billion-dollar industry based on the belief that the food we consume does not provide us with the required optimal levels of essential nutrients.

There is some truth in this; however, the 'pill for every ill' policy which the mainstream medical profession stands accused of, is fast becoming a mantra for those who push vitamin supplements. Though touted as 'natural', these supplements carry their own side-effects when the safe dosage is exceeded. They may also conflict seriously with certain prescribed medications. For example, the St John's wort herb traditionally used for anxiety, if used together with Selective Serotonin Reuptake Inhibitors (SSRIs), which are widely used anti-depressant drugs, can result in a toxic state called 'serotonin syndrome'.

One example of the beneficial use of supplements, however, can be seen in the management of premenstrual syndrome. Hormonal disruption during certain phases of the menstrual cycle causes distressing symptoms for many women, such as breast tenderness, painful periods, fluid retention, and mood changes. Vitamin B6, magnesium, evening primrose oil, chaste tree extract and indole-3-carbinol (derived from common vegetables such as broccoli), all improve these premenstrual conditions.

In some patients on high-dose statin drugs for lowering cholesterol, supplementing with coenzyme Q10 makes sense.

In such patients, the muscles tire easily with exercise and in rare cases this causes severe muscle damage (rhabdomyolysis). This is caused by the statin drugs blocking coenzyme Q10, an important energy regulator. Low coenzyme Q10 levels can cause an increase in blood pressure and a weakening of the heart muscle. Hence the value of a coenzyme Q10 supplement.

Supplements are also useful during periods of rapid growth, folic acid in pregnancy; protein supplements in proven deficiency states, during convalescence; and vitamin D for nursing home inmates, who are often short of sunlight.

A health practitioner trained in nutritional medicine can advise on the correct short-term use of supplements for specific medical conditions, or when to choose between pharmaceutical drugs and nutraceuticals (food as medicine) for benign disorders, and how to combine these for safe use.

Water

Adequate hydration is essential for healthy functioning of our bodies.

Many of us are dehydrated to some extent, not recognising our sense of thirst as we rush around in our busy lives. Our consumption of tea, coffee, alcohol and sugar-loaded beverages dehydrates us even more. Many common ailments ranging from headaches to constipation respond well to increased hydration.

Water is the essential 'fuel' enabling the detoxifying and eliminating processes in our bodies. The liver, gut and kidneys cannot perform these functions when the body is dehydrated. When toxic by-products of our metabolism are not excreted, they upset the delicate acid-alkaline balance in the body and start a cascade of biological disruption, leading to dysfunction.

How much water we should drink to stay healthy will vary with our age, activity and medications, and the seasons. The time-honoured advice of six to eight glasses of water a day will serve most adults. It is also advisable not to drink water together with food, but about twenty minutes apart from consuming food, to avoid diluting the enzymes required for adequate digestion.

For the same reason, some prefer to have water at room temperature rather than ice-cold. In towns and cities, the drinking water or tap water supplied to homes is considered safe to drink without boiling it. For sensitive individuals it may be necessary to use a reverse-osmosis filtration system if, or when, the water supply seems suspect.

Fasting

The latest thinking suggests that intermittent fasting will help us live longer.

Older Indian traditions advocated fasting from food once a month on either the new-moon or full-moon day. Longer periods of fasting may be risky to health. It is easier and safer to do a modified fast, using freshly squeezed fruit juices for the morning and vegetable juices in the afternoon, for one or two days at a time. This respite from eating cooked food rests the digestive system, especially the liver. Such respite is especially beneficial after a period of over-indulgence.

Physical Fitness and Exercise

The structure of the human body favours movement; physical activity in turn is the key to good health.

Prolonged inactivity results rapidly in muscle atrophy and joint stiffness. The World Health Organization defines fitness as:

The ability to carry out daily tasks with vigour and alertness, without undue fatigue and with ample reserve energy to enjoy leisure pursuits and meet unforeseen emergencies.

Physical fitness is associated with better digestion, weight control, improved circulation and vitality, more restful sleep, and increased feelings of wellbeing, with reduced sugar levels and muscle tension.

A fit person has a 40% better chance of surviving a heart attack than someone who is unfit.

The chief components of fitness are aerobic capacity (stamina), flexibility, and strength.

Aerobics refers to the type of exercise where oxygen is replaced as it is used up. This involves large muscle groups and needs to be sustained for at least fifteen to twenty minutes. Examples are jogging, brisk walking, swimming, cycling, skipping rope, and exercising to music. These are especially good for the heart and lungs. The improved resilience of the blood vessels results in a lower resting heart rate and lower blood pressure, with increased efficiency of oxygen exchange in the lungs. Aerobic exercise helps with weight control, speeds up the metabolism's breakdown of fat, improves muscle tone and prevents the development of arteriosclerosis or thickened arteries. The aim is to do thirty minutes of aerobic exercise at least five times a week.

Flexibility is the ability to use a muscle through its maximum range of motion without discomfort. This is achieved by stretching exercises. These can be incorporated into our daily routine, starting with a good stretch on waking before jumping out of bed, to whenever we recognise stiffness after prolonged sitting or standing, and before doing aerobic exercise. Stretching relaxes the mind, tunes the body by reducing muscle tension, improves coordination and helps prevent strain injuries. It is best done with full attention focused on the muscle being stretched while breathing in on the stretch and breathing out when relaxing. Flexibility is important when we age, as muscles weaken and joints stiffen, increasing the risk of falls.

Hatha-yoga asanas or poses improve the circulation and oxygen supply to internal organs, resulting in improved overall health. The 'sun salute' is an especially useful posture and an easy one to perform.

The patterned practices of Tai Chi and Qi Gong also incorporate gentle stretching and breathing programs suitable for all ages, with similar proven benefits.

The Alexander Technique and the Feldenkrais Method are specialised stretching techniques performed under the supervision of a trained practitioner that focus on the awareness of posture and movement. They aim to teach recognition of the interdependence of the central nervous system (thoughts and feelings) and the musculoskeletal system. Somatics is a set of exercises developed from Feldenkrais basics by Thomas Hanna and easily adapted for individual home use. I have personally found these somatic exercises helpful in managing my own injury-related back strain.

Strength is necessary for physical labour and an asset to high-level athletes. Resistance training with weights or gym machines using isometric muscle contractions increases muscle strength. This can improve bone health, and prevent or treat osteoporosis (brittle-bone disease). Maintaining muscle strength becomes important as we age: disuse atrophy or muscle-wasting can easily set in if we experience periods of prolonged immobilisation either because of injury or illness. Muscle weakness in turn affects balance, potentially causing elderly people to fall.

Each of these components of fitness is important for specific needs at different times of our lives. However, aerobic capacity is the one considered fundamental to overall fitness.

Posture is integral to how comfortable the body feels, whether at rest or during movement. Most back problems, other than those caused by injuries, are related to poor posture. They may result from increased muscle tension triggered by stress, or from inadequate exercise, awkward lifting, or even from unsupported sleeping positions on a sagging mattress. Commonly seen is lumbar lordosis or curving of the back, with the pendulous abdomen associated with obesity, weak abdominal muscles, and tight hamstrings. Similar issues arise for women who wear high heels for long periods at a time. We can only prevent back strain if we first become aware of our posture when sitting, standing, driving, watching TV, bending, kneeling, lifting or lying in bed.

There are various types of physical therapies that can help with maintaining or restoring fitness after trauma or illness. Physiotherapy and exercise physiology are useful for improving pre-operative fitness and post-operative rehabilitation. Occupational therapy and Pilates can also help in assisting recovery and improving fitness. Personal choice treatments using massage therapy, reflexology, aromatherapy, acupuncture, baths, and flotation tanks can also relieve muscle tension.

Rest and Sleep

Respite from our busy daily routines is essential for maintaining good health. Rest is easily overlooked with the unrelenting demands on our time and energy. Pausing between activities to focus on a few deep breaths and including short gaps to separate back-to-back appointments allows for breathing space, ensuring we will be ready in case one engagement runs longer than planned.

The adrenaline that drives our daytime activity can easily tip us into compulsive overdrive and interfere with our night-time sleep. We need to plan for breaks from our routine, like weekend downtime. Frequent short holidays can hold the 'wired and tired' phase at bay. This problem is magnified for shift workers whose normal day-night biorhythms are altered during night shifts.

Restful and refreshing sleep is a problem for many, from the young to the old. Too often we seek a 'quick fix' in sleeping pills rather than addressing our daytime routine and worrying thoughts. Sleep patterns are important. To understand and manage them, we need first to examine our lifestyle behaviours. Creating a relaxing routine before bedtime and avoiding TV and screen light are helpful strategies.

We secrete melatonin, a hormone which is produced in the pineal gland during exposure to sunlight in the day, to assist with night-time sleep. Adrenaline can interfere with the melatonin levels required for sleep and disrupts other key neurotransmitters essential to sleep. Too little and too much sleep can both adversely affect cognitive function. The ideal is between six to eight hours of sleep at night. Early morning wakening (between 2 and 3 am) is an early symptom of depression.

Breathing

The oxygen we breathe is vital for life. For most, breathing is usually an unconscious activity. Yet death usually results after only five minutes of complete oxygen deprivation. The brain uses 20% of the body's oxygen supply to metabolise glucose and produce energy. This same process occurs in all the cells of the body. Hence the quality of the air we breathe affects our wellbeing.

Industrial pollutants and vehicle emissions containing smog and particulate matter in our cities contribute to poor air quality and have been implicated in worsening symptoms in asthmatics. Each of us requires 3000 cubic feet of good quality air per hour to detoxify the toxins excreted by our lungs and skin. This is not a likely scenario for those working in cramped offices with poor ventilation. Most people breathe in a superficial way, with the upper part of their chest, but the complete healthy breath (abdominal or diaphragmatic breathing), has three components, starting at the upper abdomen, first filling the lower lobes of the lungs, then proceeding upwards to the middle lobes and ending in the upper chest, filling the upper lobes. This more desirable abdominal or diaphragmatic breathing is detailed below.

Hyperventilation or short rapid breathing, on the other hand, is a common feature of anxiety attacks. It washes out carbon dioxide and can cause light-headedness and chest tightness, further increasing the anxiety. The remedy is to breathe in and out of a small plastic or paper bag (sandwich size), which covers the nose and mouth. This relieves the anxiety, and the feeling of impending doom that may come with it.

Abdominal Breathing

Position: Sitting with erect back or lying flat on the back.

Sitting: Place hands over abdomen.
Imagine a balloon behind the hands.
Inflate the balloon with each in-breath.
Deflate the balloon with each out-breath.

Lying: Place hands or a light book on the abdomen. Make the hands or book rise with each in-breath, and fall with each out-breath.

Choosing Your Exercise Program

While so much has changed since I began practicing medicine, thankfully the physical body has not.

When it comes to physical health and maintenance, many fads have come and gone, and some of our messages have changed. But overall, a flexible and confident body is still the most significant benchmark of physical wellbeing.

> *We now know that a strong body feels less pain and has more flexibility, something I've said for many years.*

Why is this so? It's because a strong body gives you a nervous system that feels safe to move and needs less stiffness and resistance to protect you.

When it comes to stretching and strengthening, we know that the best routine is the one you will do. Don't confuse yourself with highly technical programs (unless that's what you really like), and know that movement is the key.

Many studies have shown that one exercise or stretching regime may be no more effective than another, but all studies show that doing something is better for your body and mind than doing nothing.

Perhaps the only real change has been a shift away from passive stretching. This term refers to where you load a muscle or muscle group, feel the stretch and then hold it for a predetermined period. Evidence has shown that this really offers little long-term benefit. Rather, the importance of dynamic stretching has come to the fore. This is not to say that incorporating some passive stretching in your warm-up or cool-down is not beneficial, only that it may no longer be enough.

Dynamic stretching occurs when you stretch the muscle with movement. Consider the athlete you might see on TV before the game, swinging their straight leg forwards and backwards. This movement through range, without too much load, and repetitively made, will do more to relax and lengthen the hamstring muscle than holding the static hamstring stretch (touching your toes).

You should also consider the effects of biological factors such as sex, age, and genetics on your body's ability and needs when trying to warm up/cool down and/or to do a daily regime targeted at maintaining health. People who are hypermobile will benefit more from strength work, compared with people who are stiffer due to genetics or age. Biological women may need different levels of load at different times of their life due to the impact of menstrual cycles and menopause and the accompanying fluctuation of their hormones.

This all brings me back to the point that you need to find what's right for you. That starts with feeling comfortable, in a program that is easy to access, and enjoyable. The key to gaining and maintaining health is repetition: as you do the exercise more, your body will adapt.

A good daily regime should include some stretching, but also focus on strength work. This can be achieved with no equipment in the comfort of your home or using whatever you have access to, including the gym or outdoor settings.

You should consider every exercise program through the lens of 'whole health'. We should understand physical health through the lens of three major aspects: cardiovascular (heart and lungs); strength and explosive (high-intensity interval training, gym and weights, rock climbing); and 'flow and restore' (Yoga, Pilates, Tai Chi). All three aspects are required for a body that is confident and strong, and fit to take on your daily tasks. When we feel sore or stiff, without any obvious injury, it's usually because one or more of these three pillars is not being maintained. Reflect on your daily or weekly (even monthly) routines and ask yourself, are you achieving a balance in all three of these areas?

If the answer is 'No', then the best place to start is gently working on the area that you are missing out on. A good approach to the body is to start with the obvious. With this approach, you should see faster results.

Most parks today will have exercise equipment dotted around them. Doing a circuit of these exercise stations every other day will yield results that you can measure simply by the increase in repetitions that you can achieve over time.

So, when it comes to a daily program, for the best results, try to focus on a full body workout, where you use the main muscle groups in the legs and arms, work through the functional ranges of the back and the spine, and combine some strength and stretching exercises. The internet is now full of people wanting to show you how to stretch and strengthen. Be careful, but also curious. If you can find a short video that you can repeat without any problems flaring up, perhaps this is a good place to start. Once you feel comfortable and your body seems to be adapting, that is the time to consider adding to your new regime.

Remember that 'slow and steady' is the key. Maintain your body and gently encourage it to adapt in the areas where it is weak, then you should feel positive changes occurring. From here, it's about setting yourself some goals and working towards them. If you are unsure, there are many professionals such as physiotherapists and exercise physiologists whom you can confidently engage to help you work through your needs and discover how to achieve your goals.

5

EMOTIONAL

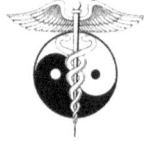

Our education system greatly neglects teaching us how to express emotions safely without being judged, ridiculed or hurt.

E motions are a given fact of our constitution, a vital aspect of our experience as living beings.

Yet expressing them remains a troublesome area for many people, with negative impact on their wellbeing. Just as expressing positive emotions can bring about a boost in energy, negative emotions can drain energy. Our education system greatly neglects teaching us how to express emotions safely without being judged, ridiculed or hurt.

Fear

Fear is the chief of all the negative emotions.

It is felt in situations which appear threatening to us, whenever we sense or anticipate danger. Often, we lose trust in our own ability to respond in such situations, and so we shrink from our fear. Withdrawing may be an appropriate response to protect oneself from immediate danger. However, such a response becomes problematic if it persists when the danger has already long passed. In such a situation, the threatened individual may needlessly remain 'on guard' just in case the threat returns. Such a person no longer feels safe and experiences the world as hostile and dangerous, fuelling more insecurity and reinforcing their need for self-protection. The most commonly felt fear is the fear of death – the great unknown, carrying the certainty of extinguishing all that is now experienced as 'me'. Many other fears haunt us – fear of illness resulting in disability, fear of losing our loved ones, fear of possible harm to our children, fear of financial disasters, fear of loss of job or status, fear of rejection or fear of being judged as inadequate...and so on.

Anger

Fear often gives rise to anger.

Anger is the expression of blocked desire. Our culture does not allow a safe way to express anger. Many of us can remember being told to be 'good boys and girls' when growing up and not to get angry. So, anger is usually suppressed when it is felt. Consequently it finds expression in uncontrolled rage, violent outbursts, and other harmful behaviours. It can morph into resentment, jealousy, blame, frustration, helplessness and depression.

Suppressed anger or rage is the emotional metaphor for physical inflammation.

Compare the description of suppressed anger in a person (red-faced and hot, muscles tight, jaw clenched, the person is about to 'explode' with fury), with the medical definition of inflammation as redness, heat, swelling and pain. The two pictures match. Inflammation is the common precursor of the onset of disease in the body. We know that changes in the physiological markers of stress (such as cortisol, the steroid hormone produced by your adrenal glands, and fibrinogen, a protein that encourages blood clotting) accompany negative emotions. Over a long period of time, these molecular changes act on vulnerable genetic tendencies to cause functional and structural disturbances to the respiratory, gastrointestinal, immune, cardiovascular, and endocrine systems. These disturbances then appear in the body as disease.

Chronic anxiety causes blood pressure to rise and the pulse rate to increase, straining the cardiovascular system. Chronic depression can suppress the immune system, increasing the risk of succumbing to infections. On the other hand, positive emotions like happiness and contentment are associated with increased output of the 'feel-good' hormones and neurotransmitters (oxytocin and dopamine), which in turn are associated with mental wellbeing.

Love

The antidote to fear is the emotion of love, in this case self-love.

Love is the unconditional acceptance of who I am, including everything that may be wrong with me – warts and all! It involves stopping self-criticism, put-down judgements, attempts to become perfect and unfavourable comparisons of oneself with others. When self-acceptance becomes unconditional, it frees up energy previously trapped in negative emotions and can boost better healing outcomes.

Where fear causes contraction and isolation, love engages with openness and connection and feeds into contentment and happiness.

Love is the most powerful healing force available to us
and needs to be consciously cultivated as a daily exercise.

When the doctor undertakes an empathetic exploration of the emotional context underlying a patient's chronic illness, this can result in the patient gaining a better understanding of the meaning behind their suffering. This process encourages the patient to consider a reinterpretation of events, bringing about changes in their behaviour – releasing blame and self-critical judgement, for example –

and helping them to embrace a more hopeful and accepting attitude. Beyond the immediate crisis of a life-challenging illness lies an opportunity for growth, achieved by first examining and understanding the role that fear-based negative belief systems have played in the process of becoming unwell.

Case Study 2: A Teenager with Acne

Beth, aged 14, came to see me with facial acne. She had tried various lotions and potions and was keen to avoid the oral antibiotics recommended by her doctor. Her mother was concerned that Beth had become reluctant to socialise and was also missing school. Beth had overheard her friends commenting about her acne in an unkind way.

I explained to Beth that the normal hormonal changes occurring at puberty had stimulated her sebaceous glands, and how the oily secretions from these had plugged the openings on her skin, causing pimples to form. I showed her an anatomical illustration of the skin and she understood that squeezing the pimples would only lead to scarring. I suggested she reduce her intake of processed foods and sugary drinks and advised her on gentle skin-cleaning strategies. I prescribed a combination of creams for the acne.

She returned a month later and was happy with her improvement. I encouraged her to continue with the treatment and addressed her self-esteem issue. I helped her to focus on her strengths – one of which was her talent in creative writing. She had already published a short story in her school magazine. She was able to identify herself as an individual who was valued for who she was, rather than being judged by her facial appearance.

Three months later Beth's acne had resolved without scarring and she had resumed an active social life with her peers.

Teenagers are at a stressful growth stage as they experience physical changes which can be challenging to their newly emerging personalities. If we merely deal with these issues at the physical level and ignore the associated emotional turmoil, we miss the opportunity to establish in the teenager a sound and healthy sense of self. In Chapter Five, we learn more about the importance of managing emotions as part of general healthcare.

One emotional reprocessing exercise my patients have found useful is called 'the forgiveness ritual'.

Forgiveness Ritual

A judgement is a held belief which is locked in place at the emotional level and cannot be changed by the conscious mind, however hard we try at the intellectual level.

These judgements may be about others or oneself, and usually relate to blame, hurt, anger or self-reproach. We see such judgements as 'truths' whenever we examine them. The energy trapped in these beliefs ('truths') becomes a block to any desired change aimed at improving our health. This trapped energy can only be accessed by ritual, because ritual bypasses the discursive ('butterfly') mind and allows emotional reprocessing and release.

The only way to release judgement is through forgiveness.

The forgiveness ritual involves writing a letter addressed to the person against whom the judgement is held, or to oneself if self-criticism is the issue. Only the author should see this letter. It should not be sent out, and the language used should not be censored for politeness or grammatical accuracy; swearwords, name-calling and scolding are all encouraged! There are three steps to this ritual:

1. *Catharsis*

The first part of the letter is the outpouring of the feelings associated with the perceived grievance – the hurt, the anger, the unfairness, the cruelty, the bullying – these are described in detail with a 'how dare you treat me this way' approach. All that one would like to say, but is unable to say face-to-face is expressed without holding back. This exercise is continued until there is nothing left unsaid about the issue and all the feelings associated with it have been expressed.

2. *'I Forgive You'*

This is the most difficult part of the ritual, where the energy must shift from the head (recounting) to the heart (releasing). It is not so hard to recount the grievance story, because we have told it to ourselves repeatedly. It is harder to forgive someone who has hurt us badly, because we feel that this forgiveness may be equated to condoning their action. But the real reason we have for forgiving them is to unburden ourselves. The 'offending' person will likely have moved on in their life without any further thought about us, but we are left still holding the negative energy of judgement. Releasing our judgement of them is not intended to condone their actions but rather to benefit ourselves, so that we can move forward. If this act of forgiveness is genuinely performed from the heart, the patient feels a huge release and a kind of lightness as the weight of judgement falls away.

3. *Disposal*

The last part of the ritual involves completing the circle by returning to the universe the energy previously held in the judgement, which is now held in the written letter. This energy originated from the universe through the actions of another or oneself. While some may choose to go the water's edge and offer the shredded pages of the letter to the ocean – our minds hold the image of water washing us clean – others may consign the letter to fire and watch it being reduced to ashes. Either way, it is gone. Yet another person may choose to dig a hole in the garden, bury the letter and plant something there, to watch it grow into something beautiful. The manner and place of disposal is a personal choice, as long as it is meaningfully done.

Case Study 3: Forgiveness Heals

Lara, who was forty-five years old, came to see me with multiple complaints that had contributed to her poor health over the last decade – migraine headaches, irritable bowel syndrome, irritable bladder, and recurrent bladder infections. Another doctor had diagnosed depression, but the medication prescribed had not suited Lara; she could not tolerate the side-effects. In the past she had her gall bladder removed for stones and her uterus removed for fibroids. She was obese. She had seen various conventional and naturopathic practitioners, but had only found temporary and minor relief for her problems each time. She appeared defeated but had not completely given up hope for improvement.

Based on the results of her blood tests, which showed a pre-diabetic state, I planned a weight-reduction diet and a walking program, encouraging her to slowly increase it to a daily brisk walk. I rationalised her long list of supplements and taught her abdominal breathing (see Chapter 4), and some basic muscle relaxation exercises. Over the next few weeks, she started to practise daily mindfulness meditation.

When I questioned her about her relationship with her ex-husband, Lara burst out crying and spilled the sorry story of a marriage marred by abuse, unhappiness and neglect. She blamed her ex-husband for destroying her health and felt very bitter towards him. Over the next few counselling sessions, I helped her to recognise how her resentment was blocking her ability to get on with her life. I suggested to her that her judgement against her ex-husband was keeping her imprisoned in her story as the victim, and that forgiveness could release her from this burden. With further encouragement and insight, she was able to write him a letter (as in the Forgiveness ritual examined in this chapter), in which she expressed her hurt and forgave him. This was not easy for her to do. She accepted some responsibility for what had gone wrong in the marriage, and from then on, she was able to forgive even herself. She started liking herself and her weight began to drop. She found a job where she felt valued, renewed neglected friendships, and started to live again.

Lara's case illustrates how our traumatised emotions and ensuing judgements can be expressed as physical complaints. Unless we explore these buried hurts, we are only putting out spot fires, and not really experiencing any lasting healing. It takes courage and trust to engage with this process. It was only when Lara relinquished resentment and blame through forgiveness that the

healing power of love could work its magic, freeing her into new
possibilities for a richer life.

Happiness

**Everyone wants happiness in their lives while equally
wanting to avoid unhappiness and suffering.**

This is a natural desire common to all of us, and we seek to
fulfil it in a material world by acquiring possessions and
manipulating events and circumstances_to suit our wants.
This may bring us temporary happiness, but this can come
at the cost of disadvantaging relationships with others.

The attempt to change the world to suit our desires and needs
potentially leads to conflict, alienation and ultimately to an
unsatisfactory and unhappy experience of life.

What we do not realise is that we are trapped by our
conditioning into reacting to the world with certain fixed
patterns of behaviour based on earlier experiences, usually
stemming from our childhood. As we grow up these
behaviours are reinforced by our parents, teachers, peers,
and culture. Our judgements of our experience as good/bad
or pleasurable/painful lead us to either desire one or avoid
the other. Invariably, if we are feeling unhappy, this creates a
need to change the 'world out there', which is blamed for
our present situation. But to deal with this scenario, what is
really required of us is an examination of our own
conditioning.

This helpful graphic on the following page shows us how life
energies representing 'the world out there', are manifested

as people, situations, and things, transmitted through our senses and then registered as our experience.

The problem for us is that we view all this through the filter or interpreter of our own addictive conditioning.

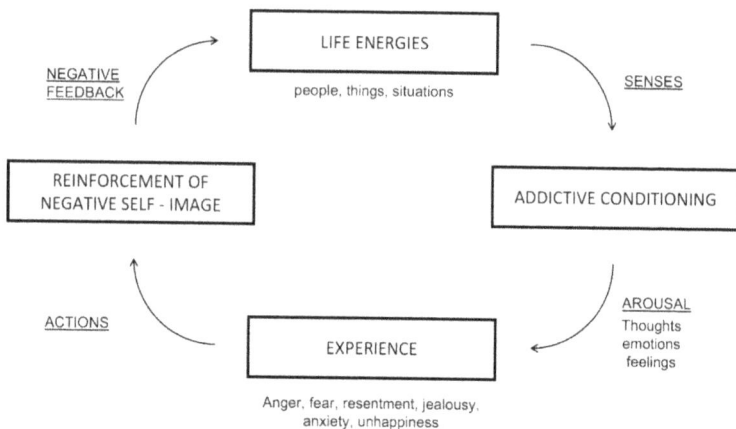

Wheel of Happiness - adapted from Ken Keyes Jr

When the situation outside us does not fit our programmed expectations, demands and desires, we experience negative thoughts and emotions, such as fear, anger, resentment and jealousy, which then cause our unhappiness.

Our actions will then reinforce our negative self-image as we criticise, blame, or reject either ourselves or others. This negative feedback that we give to people and events in our life in turn evokes an alienating and negative response from them, and so we go round the wheel again, reinforcing our belief that the outside world is really hostile and does not like us. So, we create more defences and further limit our self-expression. We spend a large part of our waking lives with our conscious thought dominated by unsatisfied desires. Our pursuit of these desires leads to a state of constant arousal and stress, resulting eventually in common psychosomatic health problems – physical illness caused by the mind.

The Wheel of Happiness

The way to change this picture into a 'wheel of happiness' is to redirect our energies into reprogramming our inner conditioning of emotion-backed demands into preferences rather than demands.

We need to stop trying to force external life energies to change. When we lovingly accept people and situations unconditionally, we begin to experience joy, pleasure, love, even reverence.

When we feed back these positive responses of unconditional love and acceptance of ourselves and of others into life through our actions and words, we can powerfully affect the life energies around us.

Now people and events start to respond positively to us and we experience increasing happiness as we go round the wheel of happiness.

Enough is Enough

We need to distinguish our needs from our wants.

This is not easy for those who are seduced by our consumer-driven culture and the attendant advertising together with social media 'influencers' who equate our happiness with more material acquisitions and ego-based power.

The stress of keeping up with the latest trends, the fear of missing out, or judging oneself as 'not good enough' creates a state of physiological hyperarousal, which impacts adversely on wellbeing and health.

Decluttering our lives of superfluous things and demands can create space for the more essential health-promoting activities for which we never seem to have enough time. A critical element of happiness is contentment once basic needs have been fulfilled. Feeling adequate and expressing gratitude for our given circumstances is to be thankful for the gift of this life and it is a feeling that will promote a positive and accepting attitude to the challenges we face. By reducing our wants and desires, and reframing them as preferences, we simplify our lives, have fewer worries, and set a more comfortable pace for ourselves, allowing us to get off the treadmill and 'smell the roses' along the way. Comparing our situation with that of others who are more disadvantaged than us can add a perspective which allows us to be grateful for our own lot.

Loneliness

Another negative influence on our wellbeing is loneliness.

This is a significant feature of our current demographic where the traditional extended family networks have been replaced by nuclear family households living separately, sometimes overseas, with limited physical contact. This was brought into harsh focus with the Covid-19 pandemic-related travel and contact restrictions imposed on us starting in about 2020. Isolation from other humans is a recognised independent risk factor affecting morbidity and mortality, especially in the older age group. As social beings we have an innate need for loving connections. Sharing and caring, helping others, can reduce self-centred selfishness and increase our own happiness. When we help someone, the 'feel good' neurochemicals in our brains increase. This is why voluntary community service work is so often recommended as a route to better mental and physical health.

Grief

Grief results from loss. The death of a loved one, significant financial loss or a forced job redundancy can all provoke grief. As an emotional reaction, it is associated with a feeling of sadness, emptiness, and deflation of energy. It is impossible to go through life without experiencing some loss-related situation. This is because of our natural attachment in close relationships, as well as our expectations of predetermined outcomes in our efforts to achieve and maintain our comfort zone. Grief becomes a problem for health if it is not processed in a timely manner. Studies have shown that unresolved grief can play a significant role in triggering many life-challenging illnesses.

In her book *Death and Dying* Dr Elisabeth Kübler-Ross highlighted the importance of understanding the grieving process associated with the death of a loved one. In my own experience with my patients, I have explained it as a four-stage sequence:

1. Denial

Denial is an immediate reflexive reaction when news of an unexpected death arrives, especially if we have only very recently seen the person in ostensibly good health. Denial is a natural response intended to protect our mental sanity from the shock of the unexpected loss. It is easier to prepare for the death of someone who is terminally ill and has been given a poor prognosis, because the mind has time to prepare for the impending loss. Denial only becomes a problem when it is prolonged into unacceptance, which can happen when there is an unexplained disappearance or a situation where death is not evidenced as a fact.

2. Reaction

This second stage is marked by the realisation that the loss we have suffered is an undeniable fact. Either we have seen the body of the deceased for ourselves, or we believe their death to be true beyond any doubt. The reaction can be a mix of emotions – a feeling of sadness accompanied by crying is only natural. We may also react with anger or blame directed against someone who we believe was responsible for our loss – the medical caregivers who could have done more to save the person's life, or the perpetrator of violence resulting in the death. We may also feel personal guilt because we feel we could have done more to prevent the death. We may feel shame if it is a case of suicide. This mix of raw emotions should be acknowledged and vented within a family circle or with supportive friends. In traditional societies there were rituals to accommodate this stage and to support the bereaved while they transitioned to the next stage. In our modern world we seem to have discounted this need and expect life to continue at its usual pace despite the experienced loss. If these emotions are suppressed, the grieving process may become prolonged, with concomitant adverse health outcomes for the bereaved. I caution my patients not to rush through this stage.

3. Acceptance

This next stage results from a realisation that continuing to discharge emotional reactions does not change the fact that the loss is final and real. A tentative acceptance sets in, and normal routine is re-established. However, whenever we remember the deceased, either by revisiting an earlier shared memory or place or event, or at times of important family gatherings like birthdays or Christmas, we will again experience a surge of emotions. It is normal for this to-and-fro experience between reaction and acceptance to continue for quite some time, until the final stage is reached.

4. Integration

In this final stage we experience a resolution of our emotions about the loss. We can remember and talk about the deceased without feeling overwhelmed. We have a perspective on our relationship from its beginning to its end along the timeline of our personal biography, seeing that we had a life before, then a life with, and now a life without that person. This stage usually starts to be felt around the time of the first anniversary of the death. We can help ourselves through this stage by enacting a ritual to mark the event and bring closure.

Grieving can be a difficult experience for someone who has had an ambivalent relationship with the deceased, as in the case of those who have been abused by a parent or close family member, resulting in estrangement. The original betrayal of trust sits uncomfortably with the need to acknowledge the loss of the biological relationship. In such a situation it helps if we can ventilate our conflicting emotions through psychological counselling. The forgiveness ritual detailed earlier in this chapter can be used as an aid to completion of this difficult grieving process.

Case Study 4: A Grieving Husband

A devoted couple, married for forty-five years, seventy-five-year-old former auctioneer Clive and his seventy-three-year-old wife Evelyn, a former nurse, had been my patients since they both retired. Clive had survived a heart attack two years earlier. He had made a good recovery and resumed an active life, playing bridge and lawn bowls and sailing his dinghy on the river once a week. Evelyn had been diagnosed with breast cancer five years earlier and had recovered from surgery and chemotherapy but had become less socially active over the past year, complaining of low-grade fatigue. The couple's only daughter lived interstate but kept in regular touch with her parents.

Evelyn tripped and fell one afternoon when Clive was out sailing. He found her slumped on the kitchen floor. She was taken by ambulance to hospital where she was found to have fractured her hip in the fall. X-rays showed the fracture was caused by bone metastasis, most likely from the earlier breast cancer. Further tests showed widespread metastases in her spine, lungs, and brain. It was decided not to operate on the fracture, and Evelyn was moved into hospice care where she died a month later.

Clive was understandably distraught and blamed himself for not being at home that fateful afternoon. I explained to him that his wife's condition was already terminal at the time of the fall, though she was remarkably functional. Her rapid decline and death had come as a shock. Clive's grief was raw and palpable. His daughter convinced him to stay with her for a month. On his return home I helped him process his loss by taking him through the stages of the grief experience, reassuring him that his anguish would recede with time. The blame that he felt was the biggest hurdle he had to surmount.

At the first anniversary of Evelyn's death, I persuaded Clive to look at the forgiveness ritual as a way to mark the event. With my gentle nudging he was able to write a letter releasing himself of the judgement he had held against himself. It took another three months for him to resume his social life.

This story of loss relates to an inevitable experience which we must all face one day. Unresolved grief has been shown to be a significant risk factor for disease, especially in the elderly. I have also witnessed how the death of a partner in a devoted and long relationship can hasten the death of the surviving spouse. This is often referred to as dying of a broken heart.

6

MENTAL

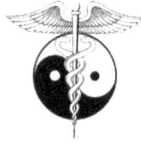

A 'positive attitude' does not mean mere fanciful and wishful thinking, but rather a determined resilience based on your trust in yourself, believing that you can marshal the capacity to meet the challenge.

The mind is a powerful force which can become a potent and positive influence on our health when harnessed correctly. Equally, chronic depression is a risk factor for a wide range of physical illnesses. What we experience as our sense of self is an interconnected system comprising thoughts (energy waves), woven together with our emotions and our physical body. The 'conversations' we have with ourselves will influence our wellbeing. In her book *Molecules of Emotion,* Candace Pert PhD, has outlined the chemical pathways in our system. Plying these pathways, neuropeptides act as messengers between our mental, emotional, and physical aspects.

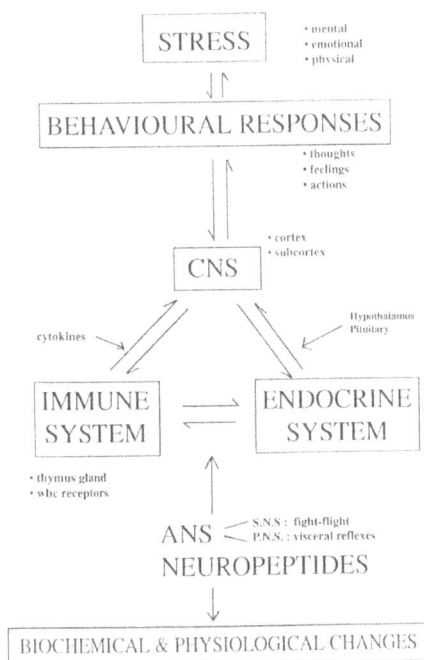

CNS: Central Nervous System. **wbc receptors:** white blood cell receptors. **ANS:** Autonomic Nervous System. **PNS:** Parasympathetic Nervous System.

The evidence that a positive mental attitude is associated with better outcomes when we are faced with a health challenge is growing. A 'positive attitude' does not mean mere fanciful and wishful thinking, but rather a determined resilience based on your trust in yourself, believing that you can marshal the capacity to meet the challenge.

Loss of trust occurs in many ways. It may result from a betrayal of trust in a significant relationship or from a prolonged period of unrelenting and apparently endless stress. The associated despondent state of mind together with a mounting sense of self-doubt, worthlessness and helplessness creates an attitude of 'give-up-itis'.

Science has acknowledged that this contraction of the vital life-force resulting from the loss of hope, is an important factor often preceding the appearance of physical illness, especially cancer. So, exploring the context of a patient's life when they are diagnosed with a serious illness can be helpful to doctors seeking to clarify the situation. Helping the patient to release their negative attitude and restore their trust in life becomes the essential first step to recovery. If a patient can reconnect with their life energy, become grounded, and feel safe and supported, this in turn will increase the recommended treatment's likelihood of success. The patient's acceptance of the situation as really happening, in the here and now, rather than denial, allows for a better considered response, and the resulting reconnection with life opens the way to positive change.

It is at this point that the doctor can augment medical management protocols by introducing effective stress management techniques as part of a personal self-care strategy.

Stress

Stress is the natural physical, emotional, and mental reaction to situations that frighten, stimulate, or excite us.

This reaction is not always negative; it may be positive (as with the release of feel-good endorphins for example). 'Eustress' is a positive reaction to a welcome and pleasurable stimulus. Distress, often accompanied by fear or anger, is a negative reaction to a challenging situation.

When we are diagnosed with a serious illness we usually take it as an existential threat and so we mount an immediate distress response. It is important for us to acknowledge this response as normal, so that we can then understand and accept the rationale for introducing into our lives, skills which will become the antidotes to counter our distress experience. Examples of these skills include Yoga, Tai Chi, Qi Gong, prayer, and meditation. Learning any of these skills and committing to their long-term practice lays a strong foundation for recovering and improving health.

Pranayama is the art of breathing according to yoga tradition. It comprises a series of specific breathing exercises meant to harmonise the flow of *prana* (vital life-energy), through the body. Regulating the breath helps to quieten the mental chatter during meditation. The breath is the mediator between the physical state and the mental state. Short, rapid and shallow breathing is associated with anxiety, whereas long, slow and deep breathing is associated with a relaxed state.

Abdominal or diaphragmatic breathing is first taught as a preliminary step to induce relaxation. Activating the diaphragm shifts the breathing from short, superficial, and rapid to long and slow deep breathing. This in turn slows down the heart rate and lowers the blood pressure.

Mindfulness and Meditation. A program of mindfulness-based meditation starts with introducing brief periods of becoming aware of the present moment by focusing attention on the sensations in the body. This is followed by teaching general muscle relaxation and mindfulness of the breath as a more formal daily practice.

Mindfulness meditation is a state of awareness centred in the present moment. It is not a passive process of mental idling, but a skill to be learnt. Once mastered, it will allow daily activities to become free of neurotic disturbances and permit a state of restful alertness. Our usual state of awareness oscillates between remembering our past with regret or remorse and imagining our future with fear or anxiety. The present moment, which is our only real chance of making any change, slips away, drowned by our mental chatter. This absent-minded state of dispersed attention, which is our 'auto-pilot' mode is an inefficient way to use our energy. This inattentiveness can result in not being alert to changes in the body which signal disease. For the practitioner, this inattentiveness can mean missing cues from the patient during consultation. Meaningful moments may pass by unnoticed and addictive patterns relating to work or pleasure can develop as habits harmful to health. Further, this lack of attention can result in accidents while driving or handling machinery. Hence the importance of training our attention to focus fully on the present moment, paying 100% attention to what is in front of us, or whatever it is we are doing, whether it be as simple as watching a beautiful sunset or washing the dishes.

The training in developing this skill, like any other learnt skill, requires commitment, regular practice, and patience. The basic requirements are simple: fifteen to thirty minutes sitting in a chair with an erect spine or cross-legged on a cushion on the floor, once or twice a day, in a quiet setting, preferably in the early morning or evening before meals.

The three characteristics of the mindfulness experience are:

1. Focusing
2. Letting be
3. Receptivity.

'Focusing' means giving your attention to a chosen restricted stimulus for an extended period. This could be your own breathing, or an image, or a mantra (repeated word or phrase). Our usually wandering 'butterfly' minds will always interrupt this process with thoughts and sensations. Joy Rains, a mindfulness practitioner, calls this 'STUFF' - Stories, Thoughts, Urges, Frustrations, Feelings. We can help ourselves in our mindfulness practice by recognising when STUFF intrudes into our awareness and then repeatedly redirecting our attention back to our chosen focus.

'Letting be' means putting aside the usual goal-directed analytical mind-state and resting in the present moment, not holding on to ideas or sensations or judging them as good or bad; being rather than doing.

'Receptivity' implies acceptance of whatever arises as happening in the here and now and as something new to be trusted, not to be feared, however uncertain, unfamiliar, or paradoxical the experience may be.

Numerous researched publications attest to the beneficial effects of meditation. Regular practice results in the reduction of stress, anxiety, depression, high blood pressure, headaches, asthma, as well as dependence on alcohol, smoking, and drugs.

There is evidence of meditation also effecting a reduction in personality disorders, aggression, and criminal behaviour. The practice improves sleep, memory, creativity, learning capabilities and motor and perceptual skills.

These effects of meditation can be seen clearly in regular meditators, manifested as demonstrated changes in the physiological levels of key stress hormones (such as adrenaline and cortisol), and neurotransmitters (such as serotonin, the 'happiness' chemical), together with an increase in alpha and theta brain waves (which indicate a state of deep relaxation), a lower metabolic rate and improved immune response. In simple terms, with meditation practice, the entire body-mind system functions in a more efficient manner, resulting in better health, harmony in relationships, and happiness.

Affirmations

Affirmations are positive statements acknowledging our innate wholeness and health. Affirmations challenge the usual negative beliefs, which dominate our conversations with ourselves and undermine our self-esteem. These negative beliefs result from criticisms we first encountered in childhood, from our parents, teachers, and influential others; later reinforced by peer groups and the surrounding culture. Comparisons with others made in a competitive context can easily cause self-doubt and ripen into an 'I am never good enough....' attitude. We then use minor setbacks or failures, which are all just part of life, to confirm the validity of this negative belief. Thus, we can become locked into a restrictive behaviour pattern marked by increasing fear, anxiety, and depression. This state of mind is a prelude to health problems.

If we want to escape from this prison of negativity, awareness is essential. We must become aware of the negative thoughts before we can challenge them. Bringing them into our consciousness and then demanding evidence of their validity is often enough to expose them as untruths. At this point it is just a matter of denying these negative thoughts any more power and dismissing them. But we may also need to immediately affirm that 'I am ok, I am alright, I am doing my best', or to make other similar positive, reassuring statements to ourselves. Affirmations can be made up to suit whichever mindset we wish to change. A general one could be 'Every day, in every way, I am feeling better'.

Negative beliefs must be challenged each time they surface and replaced with a positive affirmation. If we persist with this practice, these negative beliefs will lose their potency and weaken. Repeating affirmations strengthens our belief in them and they start to form a healthy foundation for a new sense of self. Slowly our worldview changes from 'a glass half-empty' to 'a glass half-full'. But this process will take time and patience.

Creative Visualisation and Mental Imagery

In some cases, visualisation techniques may help with recovery from intractable illness.

The mind does not distinguish between a present reality experience and the recall of a past reality experience, or even a vividly imagined imagery. When we recall past happy and enjoyable experiences the body feels the same physiological response it felt at that time, summoning into the present an increase in 'feel-good' chemicals like oxytocin and endorphins. Similarly, when we dwell on past sad, traumatic, or fearful events, our body experiences the same surge of stress hormones as it did then – adrenaline and cortisol. The 'feel-good' chemicals released strengthen the immune system while the stress hormones suppress the immune system, with obvious adverse consequences for our health.

The only precondition for successful creative visualisation is that the mind must be in a relaxed state when the positive message is given. There are two times in the day when the mind-body connection is most favourable for this – one is at the point of just slipping off into sleep, and the other is when we first awake from sleep. Visualisation done at these times has been shown to be more effective.

In his book *Centre of the Cyclone*, John Lilly said:

> *In the province of the mind, what is believed to be true is true, or becomes true, within limits to be found experientially and experimentally. These limits are further beliefs to be transcended. In the province of the mind there are no limits.*

The well-known 'placebo effect' and the less well-known 'nocebo effect' are examples of how a belief can affect physical reality. Placebo drugs, by fostering hope and positivity, can help improve the actual physical outcome, while a nocebo (a benign substance masquerading as a harmful one), by taking away hope, can cause physical harm. Hence doctors must be aware of the potential power of their spoken advice when they deal with someone who is seriously ill.

Elite-level athletes employ visualisation techniques to perfect their competitive performance. I have taught patients about to undergo surgery to visualise the entire process from beginning to end together with the desired successful outcome, and have witnessed their speedier than average recovery as a result, much to the pleasant surprise of their surgeons.

Mental imagery also helps with pain management, thus lowering the dose of strong analgesics needed to deal with chronic pain.

In my own practice I have taught patients how to raise the temperature in their hands by imagining them being immersed in a tub of warm water or being near a warming fire. For the hands to become warm, more blood must flow into them; the resulting vasodilation (dilation of the blood vessels), is not limited to the hands but is generalised in the body, leading to a lowering of blood pressure. This exercise has helped those with borderline hypertension who are not ready to embark on drug treatment. However, regular monitoring of the patient is necessary.

In his book *Getting Well Again,* Dr Carl Simonton, a radiation oncologist (cancer specialist), recounts how he successfully used mental imagery with his cancer patients by getting them to imagine their immune system cells attacking the cancer cells and destroying them.

Mental Imagery For Pain Management

Many people who have existing pain, experience the area of pain as feeling very different from other parts of the body – tight, tense, different temperature etc. The temptation is to feel you want to wall it off or push it away. This resistance only builds up more resentment and tightness. In this exercise you go into the pain, explore it, and become aware of what it really feels like:

1. Sit or lie in a symmetrical position and close your eyes.
2. Relax as completely as you can. Start progressive muscle relaxation.
3. Move your attention through the body, seeking out an area that feels different – painful, tight, under pressure.
4. Be aware of **where the pain sensation is** in your body, e.g. the tummy. Be as specific as possible, e.g. close to the skin, deep in the abdomen, in the upper or lower region. Ask yourself, 'Where is it?'
5. Be aware of **the pain's shape.** Is it like a ball, a sphere, a rod? What is its shape?
6. Be aware of **the pain's size.** How long? How wide? How deep? What is its size?
7. Be aware of **the pain's density.** Solid or light? Is it the same all the way through? What is its density?
8. What does the pain **feel like?** What is its surface texture? Is it soft and fuzzy, rough, or hard and smooth? What does it feel like?
9. What **temperature** is the pain? Hot or cold or the same as everywhere else in your body? What temperature is it?

10. What **colour** is the pain? If this is vague, imagine what colour it could be.

11. Focus on the **breath.** For three rounds of breathing, imagine drawing the breath into the body and using the breath to wash around the area of pain that you've identified. Then let the breath ebb away gently with the exhalation. For the next three rounds of breathing, imagine that the breath is drawn into the inside of the painful area to wash around the inside, then let it ebb away with the exhalation. For the final three rounds of breathing, focus on the breath again washing around the outside of the painful area, and then let it ebb away with the exhalation.

You can start all over again and repeat this 11-step body-scan, developing a very good image of the pain or sensation you are experiencing.

Humour

Humour gives us a detached perspective on our condition and helps us to shift the focus from serious preoccupation to a view of the same situation from a different perspective. We can laugh at our concerns when they are posited against the vast cosmic scale of the universe. Laughter, especially belly laughter, acts to massage the internal organs and releases endorphins. It was used successfully by author Norman Cousins to help in his own healing from a serious connective tissue disorder, as told in his book *Anatomy of An Illness.* Laughter clubs are now found in many suburbs, getting people together to laugh their way to better health. Qi Gong Master Chunyi Lin also teaches that SMILE stands for 'Start My Internal Love Engine'.

Hypnosis

In one sense it could be said that we are all acting out our lives in a hypnotic trance based on our universal consensus on reality, as we experience it through our limited human consciousness. There is good evidence that medical hypnosis is useful and beneficial in treating addictions to alcohol and smoking, as well as phobias and chronic insomnia.

By accessing and modifying subconsciously held beliefs hypnosis can free us from those habitual patterns of behaviour which negatively impact our health.

Other helpful therapies include Emotional Freedom Technique (EFT), which is a self-applied technique to counter anxiety states. Another therapy, Eye Movement Desensitisation and Reprocessing (EMDR), should only be performed with a skilled practitioner and has been shown to help in post-traumatic stress disorders. Music as therapy has also been used to great advantage in lowering high background arousal states of the sort that threaten sleep or create anxiety. 'Pet therapy' is also now in vogue in aged care homes, and for behavioural problems in children.

7

ENVIRONMENTAL

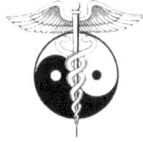

Environmental toxins arising from air pollution such as industrial smog and car exhausts, and chemical pollution from sources such as pesticides, herbicides, and microplastics are implicated in a diverse range of health problems ranging from childhood developmental disorders to adult neurodegenerative disorders.

Physical Environment

The loss of biodiversity of life on our planet is mirrored by a similar change in the human gut microbiome, which is now being linked to increasing incidence of disease in some human groups.

The United Nations Secretary General, Antonio Guterres, speaking at the COP15 Summit (15th conference of the parties to the international Convention on Biological Diversity), in December 2022, was quoted as saying that humanity has now become a weapon of mass extinction. The main drivers of this loss of species are human-induced changes in land- and sea-use, human exploitation of natural resources, global heating, pollution, and the spread of invasive species. The World Wide Fund for Nature (WWF) states in its Living Planet Index that the earth's wildlife population has decreased by 69% between 1970 and 2018, with 30% of mammals, 20% of birds and 40% of sharks and rays facing a risk of extinction.

It is now becoming obvious that human activity is impacting the complex web of life on our planet, directly affecting our own health, both as individuals and as a species. The increasing incidence of floods, bushfires, and droughts witnessed recently, together with rising sea levels, poses a great challenge to the delivery of health services to affected communities.

Environmental toxins arising from air pollution such as industrial smog and car exhausts and chemical pollution from sources such as pesticides, herbicides, and microplastics are implicated in a diverse range of health problems ranging from childhood developmental disorders to adult neurodegenerative disorders. The incidence of cancers, respiratory diseases and strokes is reportedly higher in environmentally burdened communities. Those who work in heavy industries, agriculture and construction are especially at risk. Mesothelioma (lung cancer), caused by asbestos exposure and silicosis of the lungs that affects underground miners are well established medical facts. Common sense dictates that our prolonged exposure to the cocktail of toxic chemicals that we humans experience in our environment today will have negative health consequences for us, eventually.

Nature however has a positive impact on our health. When walking by the sea, or in a forest, we are exposed to negative ions (electrically charged molecules), which have a refreshing effect on our energy systems. In contrast, the positively charged ions that we mostly encounter indoors, such as those generated by fluorescent lights in office spaces, are responsible for the sluggishness, fatigue or even depression we may feel at the end of our working day. 'Blue zones' on our planet are places where people live closer to nature, and live longer, healthier lives. City planners are now incorporating blue zones in their designs for smart cities.

Social Environment

Our social environment can also have a negative impact on our health.

The family, which on the one hand can be such a strong, safe, and nurturing space, may become a toxic space if there is neglect and/or abuse. Similarly, friendships and other close relationships can become embroiled in animosity, misunderstandings and grievances resulting in emotional turmoil and mental stress. Work, which not only provides us with an income for living, but also incorporates meaning in our lives, underpins our place in the world and gives us status in our community. Loss of financial income from lack of work, forced redundancy or long-term unemployment can have negative health consequences, with resultant maladaptive behaviour. Equally at risk is the workaholic who neglects other meaningful experiences outside their obsession with work. Workaholics find it difficult to transition into retirement, having invested their entire identity in their work role. This is why it is essential to create 'work-life balance' in our working lives. We need to recognise the difference between needs and wants, while still appreciating the value of each of the different social roles we play.

War is a particularly health-threatening environment, in both mental and physical terms. The social stress felt by those who live in communities affected by conflict and war, with ever-present danger to life and home, is enormous.

The risk of physical deprivation, with the added mental anguish of uncertainty and helplessness, saps the spirit.

Whatever the motivation for war may be, there are no winners, only loss of lives and homes on both sides; yet, despite the benefit of hindsight of two world wars in recent times, we continue to see brutal and costly wars fought even today.

Healthy Ageing

Our culture places undue emphasis on youthfulness as our most desired state. This attitude does not match the natural slowing down, which is unavoidable as we age. Of course, this is not to say that we should not stay fit by keeping physically active and taking part in activities that bring us enjoyment. But the outcome of this cultural promotion of youth is that our elders, instead of being valued for their experience and wisdom, are more commonly shunned and looked upon as decrepit and dependent. Hence the nursing home scenario of isolation and mostly (though not always) benign neglect.

One study experimented with moving nursing home residents into a resort to stay there for four weeks. They were told to dress the way they did twenty years earlier and listen to their favourite music from that time; they were given meals of their choice and encouraged to engage in socialising activities like dancing and playing games. At the end of the four weeks their blood biochemistry revealed a marked improvement in their vital health parameters. Another study has found that the health of nursing home patients improved when asked to look after a potted plant in their room.

What this tells us is that ageing is more than a merely chronological event.

Social factors which impact on meaning, connections and feeling useful have a beneficial effect on healthy ageing and need to be considered in planning for elder care. We also need more open discussions of death, so that the fear and anxiety associated with this natural event can be explored, and measures and strategies put in place to reassure the aged that their wishes will be respected.

8

SPIRITUAL

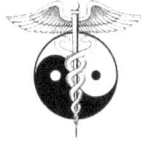

*We have all at some time in our lives felt this subtle
energy of life connecting us to something bigger and
grander than our mundane everyday existence. The
mystery of life evokes a feeling of awe and wonder and
invites our reverence.*

Let us focus now on the spiritual dimension of our being and its importance in our understanding of health, alongside the physical, emotional and mental dimensions already covered.

This is a dimension neglected by scientific medicine because it is a personal and empirical experience that cannot be scientifically validated, so far. Yet we have all at some time in our lives felt this subtle energy of life connecting us to something bigger and grander than our mundane everyday existence. When we consider the vast expanse and complexity of the universe, we cannot help but wonder about the possibility of an intelligent design, which seems to unfold with unerring regularity in the cycles of change. The process can be called 'evolution', but this does not answer the question of how or when it started. Some call the beginning of the universe 'the big bang', but then the question arises: 'What preceded the big bang?' Our limited brain capacity fails at this point. The mystery of life evokes a feeling of awe and wonder and invites our reverence.

Theistic and Secular Ethics

The theistic religions (Hinduism, Judaism, Christianity, Islam, Sikhism), posit a self-existent creator-being as the primal source and see all creation as the manifestation of this creator-being's creative energy, in all its infinite expressions.

Buddhism and Taoism do not believe in a creator-being as such but point to a 'united consciousness' – undifferentiated, eternal, and infinite – which manifests equally in all living beings and all things.

The common message of all faiths is to live a truthful life in harmony with the laws of nature. Qualities like compassion, kindness, generosity, tolerance, forgiveness, and gratitude are encouraged as inner values to be cultivated, while destructive propensities like hatred, greed, pride, malice, and bigotry are actively discouraged.

Today, as fewer and fewer people identify with organised religion, if these inner moral values are to be nurtured and preserved, they must be freed from the cultural constraints of religious dogma, and taught as universal values that can be adopted by both those who follow a faith and those who don't. These values constitute what the Dalai Lama calls 'secular ethics' – a set of basic human values, beneficial to all humanity. We all aspire to peace and happiness in our world, yet it continues to elude us. As individuals, we can start the ball rolling by cultivating healthy personal integrity. According to the Dalai Lama, the basis for such an approach rests firstly on our recognition of our shared humanity, that is, our shared aspiration to happiness and the avoidance of suffering; and, secondly, on our interdependence on each other as social beings. With this recognition we realise how our individual wellbeing is inextricably linked to that of others, and therefore we may develop a genuine concern for the welfare of others. This is the basis for a personal spirituality, which can underpin our search for meaning, purpose and satisfaction in life.

Mindfulness and Contentment

Active cultivation of these key inner values requires us to make a daily practice of awareness or mindfulness. Being fully present in the situation at hand allows us a momentary pause to reflect on the choice open to us between an automatic, conditioned reaction and a considered response. This can make the difference between perpetuating conflict or promoting harmony.

> *Tolerance and patience are the qualities called for in our times, as we rush through our increasingly frenetic lives.*

Contentment is another quality which many of us fail to develop amid the pressures of our materially acquisitive behaviour, always demanding more of whatever we think we lack. Yet when we pause to consider the difference between our needs and our wants, we begin to see how we unnecessarily create this stress for ourselves.

The Self-Serving Ego

Our recent history is replete with examples of how greed, deception and hubris lead to disasters like the global financial crisis, and these factors continue to show up in the daily news with reports of financial scams, 'pork-barrelling' in politics, and 'rorting' of public funds. When our institutions fail to show integrity, as exposed by Australia's Royal Commissions into child sexual abuse, banking, and more recently aged care, we are diminished as a society and as a nation. Betrayal of trust at this level has ramifications for the whole of our society. A self-serving attitude corrupts the moral fabric and corrodes our ideals. Self-centredness is the signature characteristic of the ego. The ego's relentless pursuit of sensate desires, security, power and control leads it into competition and conflict with others. The accompanying afflictive emotions aroused – lust, anger, greed, attachment, and pride – trap the ego into endless cycles of 'me' against 'them', perpetuating more suffering for all.

Self-Discipline and Contentment

Moderation in consumption requires self-discipline. The education system could be used initially to teach the values of restraint, tolerance, and generosity. Later, with maturity, by embracing core values such as simplicity and modesty, this practice of self-discipline becomes internalised and voluntary rather than externally imposed, and hence more enduring.

> *With this self-discipline comes a feeling of contentment and joy, which can only mean better health.*

In our rush for economic progress and material comforts too many of us have lost our reverence and respect for the process of life. Limited human understanding does not acknowledge the order behind the seeming chaos and accept that 'it is what it is.' We are always trying to control and change the life process to suit our personal preferences and wants. Modern society has lost its implicit trust in life's intrinsic order and humanity has lost its sense of the sacred.

Love and Healing

The qualities needed to connect with the sacred are innocence and humility.

We tend to judge things too much and decide how they should be, instead of holding the mind and emotions still to allow the natural expression of the life-energy – which is love. Love is the natural affinity felt by most people for each other. It is the common emotion which restores harmony in our lives. To experience this, we need to still the chattering, agitated mind through contemplation, prayer and meditation. As we disengage our awareness from the senses and the body, the background noise of our internal dialogue becomes quiet, and we experience stillness, unity and connectedness with the 'Whole'. Then our lives can reflect this deep understanding in our relationships – we don't need to dominate, possess, or try to change others; instead, we share our love with them, and this is the process that heals.

According to Victor Krivorotov, a Russian healer and mystic,

'Love is the highest form of interaction, and the prime therapeutic factor in any healing.'

It is incumbent on medical practitioners to rise to this challenge and learn to use this energy in their interactions with patients. But doctors' own spirits are often paralysed by fear, pride, arrogance and egotism. They may need to heal themselves first by practising forgiveness, relinquishing resentment, conflict and despair, as these are all obstacles to healing; they can let go of blame when they are able to forgive themselves and others. The healing power of love can move through doctors too and bring about a creative outcome only when they fully accept and take responsibility. Healing always involves restoring harmony and alignment.

The Errors of Duality and Polarisation

Beyond what we have discussed so far about the physical, emotional, mental, and spiritual aspects of health is the wider context of our human consciousness. A sense of the duality of consciousness dominates our modern human experience.

We see ourselves as separate, individual selves. The moment I identify myself as 'I', the rest of all that is 'out there' becomes 'Not-I'. This split in the united consciousness creates the illusion of two opposing aspects of reality, which are in fact complementary to each other. It limits us to only experience one of these aspects at any one time, hence excluding its opposite. From this polarised perspective we label our experiences as good-bad, pleasure-pain, accept-reject, positive-negative etc. and make our choices between these perceived options according to what seems to be in our interest. This subjective labelling is influenced by our culture and upbringing and reinforced by our experience. It rejects those thoughts and feelings which may arise, but are judged as 'not who I am' or 'not who I should be'. Thus, judged and rejected, these other aspects are buried somewhere in the subconscious, only to emerge later at a critical time amid stressed mental and physical states such as distress and disease. This buried material is referred to as 'the Shadow' in Jungian psychology.

Symptoms as Messengers

Understood from this perspective, the symptoms of illness that we may experience are not our enemies to be eliminated, but rather messengers pointing us to what is lacking in our lives and what changes are needed.

The analogy of a smoke alarm illustrates this point. When the alarm sounds we do not merely switch it off. We search for and address the source of the fire. In the same way, it does not make sense to get rid of a symptom quickly without understanding the meaning behind it and making appropriate changes in our life to address its message. Symptoms always point to an imbalance in our lives. Many of us have lost the ability to understand the language of the messenger - the symptom.

Change Consciousness Not the Body

Elida Evans wrote in her book *A Psychological Study of Cancer* **(1926): 'Cancer is a symbol, as most illness is, of something going wrong in the patient's life, a warning to him to take another road'.**

Through understanding illness in this manner, we can progress towards 'wholeness', which is what true healing is. We cannot achieve this wholeness by resisting illness. Rather we need to use the illness as an opportunity for growth and transmute it and our lives by incorporating whatever is missing. This understanding happens at the level of consciousness when it expands.

The body is neither ill nor healthy – it only reflects the patient's state and condition of consciousness.

We can see consciousness as the 'content' and the body as the 'vessel' containing it. It is the content that needs examining and changing, rather than the vessel. Merely attending to the 'vessel' is an inadequate response. It becomes clear then that we can attain the true state of health only by transcending duality/polarity and identifying with the united consciousness – reaching a state of 'At-One-ment', or 'En-Lighten-ment'.

These ideas are discussed eloquently and in more detail by Thorwald Dethlefsen and Ruediger Dahlke in their book *The Healing Power of Illness* (2016).

9

COMMON SCENARIOS

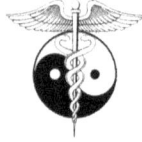

Doctors often see patients 'presenting' with evolving illnesses, which do not fit into a well-defined diagnostic category as described in medical textbooks. Doctors need to be encouraged to think 'outside the box' and apply sound clinical judgement.

The medical profession speaks of patients 'presenting' with their cases or symptoms when they seek help from doctors. Their visits are called 'presentations'.

Doctors often see patients 'presenting' with evolving illnesses which do not fit into a well-defined diagnostic category as described in medical textbooks. When challenged by this uncertainty, the litigation-conscious doctor tends to order unnecessary investigations rather than draw on their knowledge of physiology and biochemistry, which could explain the seemingly unrelated cluster of symptoms. Doctors need to be encouraged to think 'outside the box' and apply sound clinical judgement in such situations.

Below I briefly discuss common conditions that I have encountered in my own medical practice:

Functional Hypoglycaemia

Patients often report energy dips around mid-morning and mid-afternoon. They only rarely recognise this issue's relationship with eating habits; they usually mask their condition with morning and afternoon tea-breaks (caffeine and sweet snacks).

When questioned they may admit to sugar cravings. Accompanying symptoms may include faintness, mood swings, irritability, palpitations, anxiety and disturbed sleep. When people consume refined carbohydrates, which high in sugar, the pancreas produces insulin in response to the resulting high blood sugar levels – insulin is a protein hormone that regulates the body's sugar levels.

The insulin then clears the sugar from the blood and sends it for storage in the liver and muscles as glycogen, ready to be converted into the sugar glucose for future physical energy needs. This sudden drop in blood sugar levels is first registered by the brain, which depends on sugar as its energy source; the adrenal glands then pick up the alarm signal sent by the brain and respond by secreting adrenaline. This results in conversion of the glycogen to glucose, to feed the brain.

At the same time, the person becomes aware of the need to eat something quickly and they respond by eating whatever is at hand – usually a sugary snack. This provides instant relief, but now we again have a high blood sugar level which provokes insulin secretion, and so the whole cycle starts again. The chart on the following page shows this 'cycle of woe' clearly. The interval between the energy dips is usually about three hours. During the dip (hypoglycaemia), the person experiences brain fog and feels tired and drowsy; during the sugar high they can also feel the effects of the adrenaline – patients report feeling 'charged', anxious and tremulous. Caffeine, which mimics the effects of adrenaline, only adds to these symptoms.

If we do not recognise and correct this physiological upheaval, it will eventually result in relative insulin depletion and increased risk of developing insulin resistance and mature-onset diabetes. The adrenal glands may also be unable to keep up with the increased demand on them, resulting in a state of lowered energy and drive.

The way to correct this dysfunctional state is to eliminate all refined carbohydrate snacks, sugar, and caffeine from the person's diet and introduce a three-hourly pattern of eating protein or complex carbohydrate snacks.

Hypoglycaemia – Cycle of Woe

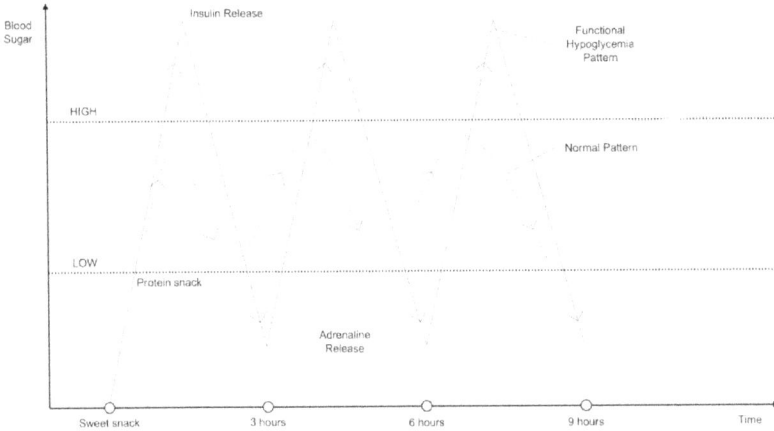

This results in the gentler rise and fall of blood sugar levels required for homeostasis (physiological balance), with reduced insulin and adrenaline secretion. This process will resolve the patient's symptoms.

Supplements like alpha-lipoic acid (a natural antioxidant that can attack the dangerous free-radical waste created when the body converts food to energy and so assists in converting glucose into energy), selenium, chromium, and zinc can also help to sensitise insulin receptors and improve metabolic function.

Stressed individuals are more prone to this condition; medical practitioners often mistakenly attribute the symptoms to neurosis, leading to the inappropriate prescription of tranquilliser medication.

Case Study 5: A Stressed Young Mother

June, a twenty-nine-year-old mother of two toddlers, came to see me with palpitations, insomnia, headaches, panic attacks and agoraphobia (fear of open spaces and 'the outside'). Her husband's work took him away from home for two weeks at a time. She ventilated her feelings and admitted that she was not coping. She was reluctant to take the tranquilliser medication prescribed for her, as she wanted to be alert to the needs of her young children.

I explained to her how her anxiety symptoms were caused by her hyper-aroused state and how her energy crashes could be related to a low blood sugar level - functional hypoglycaemia.

She was resorting to coffee and sweets mid-morning and mid-afternoon 'to keep going'. I suggested she reduce her caffeine and processed food intake, while aiming to substitute these with protein-based snacks, and not miss meals. She agreed to set aside some time in the day for home-based gentle stretching exercises and to start Vitamin B complex and magnesium tablets.

I taught her abdominal breathing, and suggested she practise the calming 'Coming to our senses' exercise, at least a few times a day. She was well motivated and the following week I was able to introduce her to general muscle relaxation and to the relaxation response. She practised these exercises twice a day and returned two weeks later reporting better sleep, no palpitations or headaches, and feeling panicky only when she became frantic. By the following month she was pacing herself much better, taking her kids to the park, and was also helping in the local playgroup.

It is not uncommon for someone like June to confuse self-care with selfishness. Driven by the demands of our responsibilities to family and work, we can easily neglect our own health needs. Yet we cannot fulfil these very same responsibilities when we ourselves are not well. The other relevant point to emphasise is that the motivation to practise relaxation techniques is a prerequisite. As with learning any new skill, regular practice also brings results. The physiological changes accompanying relaxation manifest in improved coping behaviour.

Coming to Our Senses

A quick relaxation and awareness technique

Become aware of:
Touch: The feel of the clothes touching your body.
Buttocks: Pressing against the seat of the chair.
Feet: Touching the floor.
Face: Air brushing across it.
Taste: Residual taste of any food consumed earlier.
Smell: Ambient smells in the immediate environment.
Sight: Eyes open – see the objects in the field of vision.
Eyes closed – see the shapes in the patterns of light and darkness.
Hearing: Listen for nearby sounds, and then for faraway sounds.

Candidiasis

Chronic infection with the yeast Candida is another common underlying cause for poor health that conventional doctors seldom recognise.

The impact of this condition is greater than just the oral and vaginal thrush (fungal infection of areas like the mouth and vagina), that is often triggered by using oral antibiotics and the contraceptive pill. If the immune system has been compromised, by using immunosuppressive drugs for example, this will make the body more vulnerable to such infections. Similar vulnerability arises from the depletion of the friendly microflora (living microorganisms), in the gut induced by long-term use of broad-spectrum (multi-target), antibiotics - for acne, for example - and oral steroids. A diet rich in yeast and refined carbohydrates feeds the fungal candida yeast, encouraging its overgrowth.

A wide range of disorders from neuropsychiatric (depression, anxiety, irritability); digestive (irritable bowel syndrome [IBS]); allergies (skin rashes and nasal congestion); and hormonal (premenstrual syndrome, impaired sex drive and function), to fatigue and generally feeling unwell, will improve if the underlying chronic yeast infection is detected and treated. Children who have been treated with repeated courses of antibiotics for recurrent colds or middle-ear infections may develop yeast-connected health problems like irritable behaviour and learning difficulties, together with digestive, respiratory, and skin disorders.

An extreme example of yeast overgrowth in the gut is the 'auto-brewery syndrome'. The fermentation of sugars by yeast in the gut produces alcohol. The patient then presents with all the signs of alcohol intoxication.

Treatment starts with eliminating all refined carbohydrates and yeasty foods for one week, followed by oral Nystatin (an anti-fungal medication) for at least two weeks to reduce the overgrowth of infection in the gut reservoir. When the symptoms start to improve, the patient should continue with the carbohydrate-free diet in a modified way. Adding a probiotic or yoghurt to the diet helps to replenish the gut microbiome; supplementing with yeast-free vitamin B complex, vitamin C and essential fatty acids is also beneficial.

Case Study 6: A Child with Glue Ear

Two parents, both well-informed professionals brought Amy, their four-year-old, to see me.

She was their first child, delivered by caesarean section because of a breech presentation at birth (the reverse of normal head-first childbirth, with the lower body arriving first). There had been problems with breast-feeding when her mother, Jane, developed mastitis. With the duly substituted cow's milk formula, Amy developed colic and became unsettled. A middle-ear infection was diagnosed at age two, and she had been given repeated doses of antibiotics for recurrences. Oral thrush and nappy rashes accompanied these infections. Their GP had referred them to an ear, nose and throat (ENT) specialist who had documented mild hearing impairment and recommended a grommet (a small ventilation tube), to be inserted in the ear to drain fluid accumulation. The parents were keen to avoid this intervention, so they sought my advice.

I explained to them with the aid of anatomical charts how the fluid that had accumulated in the eustachian tube that connects the middle ear with the nasal-sinus cavity had become viscous with recurrent infections. This fluid was now thick enough to prevent the eardrum from vibrating freely in response to sounds as it should - a condition called 'glue ear'.

I also explained to them that repeated doses of antibiotics had altered Amy's gut flora, favouring an overgrowth of yeast, as evidenced by the oral thrush and nappy rashes. The parents agreed to trial a diet free of yeasts, sugars, dairy and preservatives. (See 'Low Stress Diet' chart in Chapter Four). I prescribed oral Nystatin for two weeks, liquid Bisolvon to break up the mucus (Bisolvon being a mucolytic drug), and a lactose-free probiotic. Amy was also taught the 'Valsalva manoeuvre' (blowing up a balloon to unclog the ears) which she thought was fun. She also agreed to allow her mum to instil a saline solution up her nose twice a day.

Two weeks later, Amy's parents reported that her noisy breathing at night had resolved, her appetite had improved, and she now had daily formed stools with no more abdominal pains. When repeated eight weeks later, Amy's audiogram showed normal hearing, and the ENT specialist was no longer insisting on surgery. Both Amy and her parents were happy with the outcome.

This case illustrates how a common case can be managed by well-motivated supportive parents who have been given full explanations and practical advice. If they act on this advice, their actions can then delay, or possibly avoid further intervention. I have also found that children who are fussy eaters, even as young as Amy, will cooperate to change their diet if the change makes them feel better.

Gut Issues – SIBO/SIFO/IBS

Small intestine bacterial overgrowth (SIBO), small intestine fungal overgrowth (SIFO), and irritable bowel syndrome (IBS) are overlapping dysfunctions of the gut, presenting with bloating, constipation/diarrhoea, painful colic, burping/flatulence, heartburn and nausea.

The accompanying malabsorption of nutrition can result in deficiencies of iron, vitamin B12, vitamin A and vitamin D. The common offending food triggers for such conditions are gluten, dairy, yeast, and sweets. In the background is a disturbed balance of gut flora, often from prolonged antibiotics, and inadequately treated episodes of gastroenteritis, or impaired digestive enzyme secretions. Inflammation of the protective gut lining by infective agents causes increased intestinal permeability, sometimes called 'leaky gut syndrome', and consequent food sensitivities. Weight loss or blood in the stools are 'red flag' symptoms and should prompt investigations to exclude inflammatory bowel disease (IBD) or malignancy such as cancer. Polymerase chain reaction (PCR) testing of stools of infective agents can help in targeting the correct therapy. I have seen cases in which the microscopic Blastocystis parasite was the culprit organism, ingested from contaminated rainwater tanks in infrequently visited holiday houses in south-western Australia. Gut infections acquired overseas and inadequately treated can also result in lingering gut problems. Infection with the Giardia parasite is another common cause. Treatment of many gut problems involves excluding the trigger foods: for example, the 'FODMAPS' diet can be trialled – this relates to the exclusion of fermentable oligosaccharides, disaccharides, monosaccharides and polyols, all naturally occurring sugars that may not be properly absorbed in the small intestine and are therefore implicated in IBS cases. Alongside the exclusion of specific foods, the judicious use of anti-microbial herbs, digestive enzymes, and probiotics can also help the gut lining to recover from inflammation. As always, stress equally plays a big part through the now much-discussed gut-brain axis and needs to be addressed.

Challenging Conundrums – CFS/MCS/FM

Chronic fatigue syndrome (CFS), multiple chemical sensitivity (MCS) and fibromyalgia (FM), a painful musculo-skeletal disorder, comprise a group of not fully understood illnesses that present a challenge to the primary care doctor.

The trigger for their onset is either a viral or bacterial infection (the Epstein-Barr virus and herpes viruses have been implicated), exposure to organophosphorus (organic chemicals derived from phosphoric acids, e.g., Malathion) and carbamate pesticides (Baygon, for example); or physical and/or psychological trauma in the case of fibromyalgia. Genetic, hormonal, and nutritional factors may make a patient more susceptible to these conditions, so these factors should also be considered. These illnesses cause chronic multi-system poor health that can last for years. Patients commonly tire easily and complain that they can get little relief even after rest or sleep. In the case of CFS, the other common symptoms are impaired memory or concentration, sore throat, tender lymph nodes, muscle pains, multi-joint pains and headaches.

Despite more than thirty years of research we are still not certain how these conditions originate or develop. One hypothesis suggests that the initial trigger leads to a vicious cycle of increasing levels of the free radical nitric oxide and the oxidant peroxynitrite, which are responsible for disrupting energy production at the mitochondrial (cellular) level, stimulating an excess of free radicals. This 'free radical storm' then provokes inflammation. This damaging process causes what we call 'oxidative stress', damaging cells and DNA, even contributing to ageing.

A whole-person approach involving a compassionate and flexible attitude is required to help these patients, who typically have a patchy pattern of improvements interspersed with periodic setbacks. They need a low-stress diet that eliminates reactive foods. Certain supplements have been shown to aid recovery: intravenous vitamin C, intramuscular vitamin B complex, glutathione, the fat oxidiser carnitine, magnesium and anti-oxidants. Some preliminary studies show that low-dose Naltrexone (a prescription drug best known for its control of opioid or alcohol craving, as well as anxiety) may relieve the troublesome symptoms these patients experience. Carefully graduated stretching and aerobic exercises supervised by an exercise physiologist, together with mindfulness training, can complement their recovery program.

Temporomandibular Joint Dysfunction

The temporomandibular joints (TMJs) at the junction of the skull and the jawbone mark an area of the body where

many people hold increased muscle tension arising from stress.

Clenching of the facial muscles is a common reaction to unexpressed rage or anger; similar is the bruxism (teeth-grinding), that can occur during sleep. Symptoms ranging from headaches to jaw pain and facial pain result from compression of the articular disc, enabling smooth joint movements. In severe cases the disc may even dislocate partially or wholly, causing a 'lockjaw' situation. Patients who present with ear pain and have no sign of infection in the ear will show tenderness around the TMJ. The examining doctor can observe the patient's limited ability to open the mouth, and sometimes there will also be a clicking sound to the jaw movement. The pain referred from the TMJ sites often covers the head, neck, face, and throat areas owing to the multiple muscles involved in moving the TMJs.

Multiple and varied symptoms may all result from TMJ dysfunction, as can be seen in the itemised list below. Primary care practitioners often miss the diagnosis of this problem, an omission which can lead to unnecessary investigations and tests. Commonly, a dentist will diagnose the disorder from the patient's ground-down molars.

Headaches/Head pain
Forehead & Temple
Migraine
Sinus pain
Hair and scalp painful to touch

Mouth
Discomfort
Limited opening of mouth

Jaw clicks shut or open
Jaw deviates to one side when opening
Inability to smoothly articulate
Can't find bite

Teeth
Clenching & grinding at night
Looseness & soreness of back teeth

Jaw
Clicking/popping jaw joints
Grating sounds
Pain in cheek muscles
Uncontrollable jaw/tongue movements

Throat
Swallowing difficulties
Sore throat, with infection
Laryngitis, voice irregularities/changes
Coughing or clearing of throat
Constant feeling of foreign object

Ears
Hissing, buzzing or ringing
Decreased hearing
Ear pain/earache, without infection

Neck
Lack of mobility, stiffness
Neck pain
Tired sore muscles
Shoulder aches & backaches
Arm & finger numbness/pain

Eyes
Pain behind eyes
Bloodshot eyes
Bulging eyes
Sensitive to sunlight.

The doctor should give the patient a reassuring explanation of the causes, advise them to practise awareness of jaw-clenching during the day and also teach them simple muscle-stretching exercises to relieve the pressure on the joint disc. In severe cases a TMJ splint can be used at night to protect the disc from compression due to unconscious clenching during sleep.

Biomechanical Foot Problems

Pronation - rolling over of the feet - presenting as functional flat feet, is a common but often overlooked cause of multiple foot, knee, and back complaints:

Plantar fasciitis, presenting as heel pain, is caused by the stretching of the ligaments running from the heel to the toes. The traction on the heel bone may result in a bony growth called a 'spur'.

Achilles tendonitis is an inflammation of the tendon in which traction acts on and inflames the Achilles tendon at the back of the heel.

Metatarsalgia presenting as ball of foot pain, causes a burning sensation in the front part of the foot. It can cause callus formation and progress to 'Morton's neuroma' where entrapment of the interdigital nerves leading to the toes can cause numbness, tingling and pain.

Bunions are bony lumps which form on the big toe joint from a combination of genetic factors and frequent rolling of the foot that puts excess weight over the big toe joint when walking.

Shin splints present as tired, aching legs, caused by straining and stretching of the calf muscles and ligaments along the shins.

Patello-femoral knee pain - referring to the kneecap and thigh - is easily treated, but because the feet are often not checked for fallen medial arches, this pain is often diagnosed as caused by arthritis. Such misdiagnosis leads to unnecessary investigations and treatments. This condition in fact results from an internal rotation of the tibia (lower leg) that exerts force on the patella (kneecap), causing it to track out of its normal groove. Correcting this misalignment can prevent excess wear and strain on the menisci (cartilage cushions of the knees). Failure to correct it will ultimately lead to degenerative changes that may eventually require surgery.

Iliotibial band (ITB) syndrome - referring to the hip and leg - presents as pain on the outside of a knee joint and on the outside of the hip. It is caused by abnormal friction or rubbing of the supportive fibrous iliotibial band that runs between the knee and hip joints. This condition again results from the internal rotation of the legs.

Lumbo-sacral (lower back pain) manifests in the back where the sacrum connects the spine to the pelvis, as a result of lordosis (curvature) of the lumbar or lower-back spine: as the feet roll over and the legs internally rotate, the pelvis is forced to tilt forward, resulting in increased tightness and stiffness of the lower back muscles and increased spinal curvature.

All the above conditions result from functional flat feet. They can be managed by correcting the biomechanical alignment of the feet with simple off-the-shelf medial-arch orthotic supports or custom-made inserts fitted by a podiatrist or sports medicine doctor. A physiotherapist can advise on the correct stretching exercises.

10

CANCER

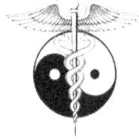

By not feeling alone, knowing that there were others in a similar situation, learning from one another in a positive and supportive atmosphere, and by ventilating their distress while feeling safe from judgement, my patients could discover meaning in their suffering and use their health crisis as an opportunity for personal growth.

P roviding continuing support and care for patients newly diagnosed with cancer is a challenge in primary care practice. My approach has been to first give the patient a simplified explanation of how cancer can develop at the cellular level from changes to the normal cell going through the stages of atypia (subtle shifts away from normal), then abnormality, followed finally by cancer. Genetic tendencies as well as immune dysfunction resulting from stress, both influence this process in its onset as well as its progression.

The Role of Antioxidants

Oxidation is the biochemical driver of inflammation, hence the beneficial role of antioxidants in checking and possibly reversing this process. The five main antioxidants that the immune system needs for its best function are vitamins A, C and E, and zinc and selenium. These can be used as a supplement together with whatever is the chosen form of medical therapy – chemotherapy, radiation therapy or surgery. Anecdotally, intravenous vitamin C given weekly at doses of fifteen to thirty grams has helped cancer patients deal better with the toxic side-effects of medical therapy.

Diet

A predominantly plant-based diet is the optimal way to obtain essential nutrients. Reducing or avoiding carcinogenic foods like processed meats, which are high in nitrates, is essential, especially for bowel cancers. Eliminating fatty foods and foods high in gluten and sugars certainly reduces the inflammatory burden, which impairs immune function.

The Role of Stress

When we talk about stress and cancer, we are not referring to the usual day-to-day stresses we all face. The stress that really counts in triggering cancer results from either a single major event in the person's recent life or a series of minor events, each succeeding the previous one in an unrelenting way. These stresses can range from physical to emotional trauma, significant loss (financial, job, relationships), or unresolved grief from which the patient has never fully recovered. Cancer patients may also present with the associated experience of helplessness or hopelessness (give-up-itis'). Such significant life-changes precede the cancer diagnosis in many cases. It is important for the doctor to elicit this history from the patient so that attention can be focused on the resolution of such issues as far as possible, as an essential part of the healing journey.

The Importance of Self-Care

The doctor then gives the cancer patient an outline of a self-care program – physical, emotional, mental and spiritual – to consider as their personal response and responsibility, to complement the medical treatment their specialists have prescribed for them.

Positive Attitude

In subsequent sessions with the patient, I usually address specific issues which they wish to explore and introduce relaxation techniques and visualisation exercises. I share with them the research evidence for adopting a healthy lifestyle and maintaining a positive attitude, while trying to find meaning in their suffering. When researchers have followed up on cancer patients who remain unexpectedly still alive against all the odds, despite being given a very poor prognosis at the time of their diagnosis, they have found some common attitudes that characterise this survivor group, summarised here as the 'Four Cs'. These beneficial attitudes and life-changes can result in not merely surviving but also thriving:

1. Challenge

The doctor must encourage their patient to consider the diagnosis as a challenge rather than a 'done deal' of poor prognosis. Adopting a positive attitude and feeling empowered releases energy for planning a considered response, as opposed to a contraction fuelled by fear and insecurity. It is important to recognise that hope and trust in a positive outcome should never be negated, however apparently dismal the situation. In many patients the response to treatment is unpredictable, and taking hope away from them could be the death-knell for any who are struggling with their condition. The 'nocebo' effect is just as powerful in its negative effect on recovery as the placebo effect is positive.

2. Control

The doctor should encourage their cancer patient to take control of the situation, get expert opinions on therapy, discuss the options but stay in charge of the decision-making process, and not be bullied by fear-mongering others - be they specialists or family members. No good outcome can result from the patient going along with a proposed therapy when they do not really feel it is their personal choice, but merely a position they have adopted chiefly to please 'significant others'. These decisions can become a daunting exercise for the patient faced with a plethora of choices of treatment following the shock of the diagnosis, so it is advisable for the doctor and family/friends to adopt a respectful and patient approach.

3. Commitment

Those cancer patients who flit about in search of a 'magic' cure, sometimes travelling overseas for unproven treatments, do not do as well as those who take responsibility and stay committed to a self-care program based on the sound evidence of good health habits which are applied consistently and daily. Even small changes to diet and exercise, and rearranging priorities in favour of healing relationships and reducing stress, can go a long way towards promoting healing if practised in a sustained way, as a life-change.

4. Connectedness

This is just another word for love. Those cancer patients who have a loving and supportive network of therapists, family, friends, and community do much better than those who feel isolated and alone with their challenge.

For many years I ran a cancer support group for my patients based on the evidence that such groups foster an improved outcome, not only in terms of better survival statistics, but also in terms of improved quality of life. By not feeling alone, knowing that there were others in a similar situation, learning from one another in a positive and supportive atmosphere, and by ventilating their distress while feeling safe from judgement, my patients could discover meaning in their suffering and use their health crisis as an opportunity for personal growth.

Epigenetics

This new science explains that the genes we inherit are only a blueprint, and do not alone determine whether we will experience cancer. 'Epi' means 'above and beyond', implying some other influences above and beyond the blueprint can initiate or mediate changes in the body, which are expressed at the cellular level and may manifest as cancer. This 'above' is also consciousness – our belief system, our world view. How we interpret or perceive 'the world out there' affects our responses and behaviours. Stress experienced from life challenges such as trauma, loss, grief, etc. has its emotional correlates – fear, anxiety, depression, anger, hopelessness, helplessness – and accompanying physico-chemical changes which promote inflammation and impaired immunity in the body.

The conclusion is that we do not have to be fatalistic and live in fear of getting a cancer just because it runs in the family. Attention to a healthy lifestyle can attenuate or even override this genetic tendency.

11

BEYOND PHARMACEUTICALS

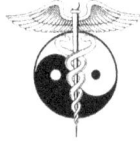

My hope is that more health practitioners will consider and embrace the wider responsibilities of their role as teachers of health to their patients, rather than be reduced to the soul-destroying practice of disease management with pharmaceuticals alone.

The complexity of illness demands that we expand the scope of our attention in this way if we are to be effective doctors.

The Doctor-Patient Partnership

Having considered the influences on health from the physical, emotional, mental, environmental and spiritual perspectives, we can conclude that there is much that the individual person can do to help improve their health by adopting simple health habits in each of these domains. Of course, working with an empathic health practitioner is a great advantage in terms of the continuing support and guidance, which can be helpful in staying the course, especially when confronted by the challenges of a chronic illness.

My hope is that more health practitioners will consider and embrace the wider responsibilities of their role as teachers of health to their patients, rather than be reduced to the soul-destroying practice of disease management with pharmaceuticals alone. The complexity of illness demands that we expand the scope of our attention in this way if we are to be effective doctors.

Patient Self-Care

The patient too must take more responsibility for self-care, by adopting healthy personal lifestyle changes. They should not become just a passive recipient of medical care expecting the doctor alone to 'fix' the problem. Much more could be said about the parlous state of our so-called health services, but this is not my brief in this book.

We've Been Here Before

The ten keys to good health attributed to the ancient Greek philosopher-scientist Pythagoras, which I have listed below, serve to remind us that we do not need to reinvent the wheel but only to use it well!

There is nothing new under the sun.

— PYTHAGORAS

1. Silence and meditation.
2. Mnemonics - memory and awareness.
3. Temperance - moderation in all things.
4. Fortitude - strength and courage.
5. Philanthropy - love, compassion and friendship.
6. Erudition - learning, especially about one's environment.
7. Music - all aspects of harmony.
8. Dietetics and fasting - the essence of health.
9. Exercise and activity - for flexibility and vitality.
10. Method, order and efficiency.

SUGGESTED FURTHER READING

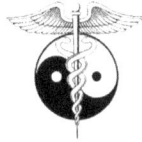

I have included below an eclectic list of books from my personal library that I have found useful in developing and grounding my understanding of the wider ramifications of healthcare.

There is so much information on self-care out there that readers need to be quite discerning to avoid being led astray by dubious claims being made about unproven and expensive programs:

Juice Fasting: Dr Paavo Airola

by Daniel G. Amen MD:

Change your Brain, Change your Life
Healing the Hardware of the Soul

Creative Meditation and Multidimensional Consciousness: Lama Anagarika Govinda

Diet and Nutrition: Rudolf Ballentine MD

The Power of the Mind to Heal: Joan Borysenko & Miroslav Borysenko

Healing your Feelings: Greg Brice

Joy's Way: W. Brugh Joy MD

Food Chemical Sensitivity: Robert Buist PhD

My Big TOE: Thomas Campbell

The Healing Power of Illness: Thorwald Dethlefsen and Ruediger Dahlke MD

Beyond Religion: His Holiness The Dalai Lama

The Emotional Life of Your Brain: Richard Davidson

Meditation as Medicine: Dharma Singh Khalsa MD and Cameron Stauth

by Norman Doidge MD:

The Brain that Changes Itself
The Brain's Way of Healing

by Larry Dossey MD:

Beyond Illness
Recovering the Soul

by Masaru Emoto:

The True Power of Water
The Healing Power of Water

Anthroposophical Medicine: Dr Michael Evans & Iain Rodger

Breathing Alive: Reshad Field

Man's Search for Meaning: Viktor Frankl MD

Vibrational Medicine: Richard Gerber MD

Wellbeing Matters: David Gore & Inge Benda

Spiritual Emergency: Stanislav Grof MD

Letting Go: David R. Hawkins MD PhD

Stress, Distress, and Illness: Dr Ian Hislop

Food For Naught: Ross Hume Hall

Inner Work: Robert A. Johnson

Full Catastrophe Living: Jon Kabat-Zinn

Handbook to Higher Consciousness: Ken Keyes Jr

The Way to Vibrant Health: Alexander Lowen MD & Leslie Lowen

Spiritual and Mental Healing: MacDonald-Bayne

Listening to the Body: Master & Houston

You and Stress: Dr Bob Montgomery & Lynette Evans

Care of the Soul: Thomas Moore

The Power of Your Subconscious Mind: Joseph Murphy

by Dr Dean Ornish:

Dr Dean Ornish's Program for Reversing Heart Disease
Love and Survival

Explaining Unexplained Illnesses: Martin L. Pall PhD

Denial of the Soul: Scott Peck

Mind as Healer: Kenneth R. Pelletier

Happiness: Matthieu Ricard

A Practical Guide to Holistic Health: Swami Rama

Healing the Healer: Rama Kirn Singh Khalsa

Soul Medicine: Norman Sheely & Dawson Church

Peace, Love and Healing: Bernie Siegel MD

The Secret Life of Your Cells: Robert B. Stone

by Eckhart Tolle:

The Power of Now
Practising The Power of Now
Stillness Speaks
The New Earth

The Science and Art of Healing: Ralph Twentyman

Health and Healing: Andrew Weil MD

Integral Life Practice: Ken Wilber, Terry Patten, Adam Leonard, & Marco Morelli

Soul Stories: Gary Zukav.

ACKNOWLEDGEMENTS

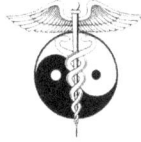

Little did I realise the complexity of bringing this book to birth. The easiest part was writing it, then came the realisation that I needed help in producing it.

The following are some of the people who have helped me in this process, without whom this would have remained an unfinished project.

Professor Avni Sali, for kindly and without hesitation agreeing to provide the Foreword to the book. I appreciate him as a mentor who has been at the forefront of promoting Integrative Medicine not only in Australia, but internationally.

Ilsa Sharp, my Editor and old friend, whose meticulous yet sympathetic editing has transformed my manuscript into this very readable book that you hold.

Hardeep Singh, for his help in laying out the initial format of the book.

Manjit Kour, for her copy-editing of the first draft of the manuscript.

Roshan Singh, Physiotherapist at A Fine Balance Physiotherapy, for his contribution to the section on Physical Fitness and Exercise.

Marian Cross, for rescuing me on many occasions from the roadblocks I encountered with my rudimentary computing skills.

Andra and Imants Kins for reading through the first transcript and for their valuable suggestions.

Michelle Simone, Chief of Staff, and her team at Hill of Content Publishers, for not only believing in the value of my book's message, but also for their professional yet empathic management of the whole process of delivering this book in the excellent format that you now hold in your hands.

And, finally, all my patients who have shared their life stories with me over many years, trusting in me for support and guidance, and from whom I have learned much about resilience in the face of suffering.

GLOSSARY

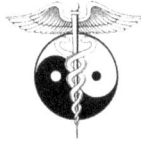

Adrenaline: hormone secreted by the adrenal gland in response to strong emotions such as excitement, fear, or anger. It causes the heart rate to increase and charges the body with energy.

Alpha brain waves: produced by the brain when a person is in a relaxed and calm state, e.g., during meditation.

Allopathic: the medical model based on treating disease by conventional means, i.e. with pharmacological drugs, surgery, and radiation therapies.

Alkaloids: organic molecules found in certain plants, fungi and bacteria that are potentially toxic to humans.

Alpha-lipoic Acid: antioxidant found in foods (red meat, carrots, beets, spinach, broccoli, and potatoes) which breaks down carbohydrates and increases energy.

Amino-acids: organic compounds incorporated into proteins.

Analgesic: pain relieving medication.

Anorexia: eating disorder with restricted food intake causing weight loss, typically accompanied by a disturbed perception of body weight and image.

Antigen: a toxin or foreign substance which induces an immune response in the body, especially the production of antibodies.

Antibody: a blood protein produced in response to and counteracting an antigen.

Antioxidant:

a) a substance inhibiting oxidation, used to counteract deterioration of stored food products.

b) a substance such as Vitamin C or E that removes potentially damaging oxidising agents in the body.

Arteriosclerosis: thickening and hardening of the walls of arteries, compromising blood flow.

Articular disc: cartilage plate found in joints, allowing for smooth movement.

Atypia: earliest structural abnormality in a cell which could indicate likely pre-cancerous progression.

Atomists: Ancient Greek philosophical school postulating that the physical universe is composed of fundamental indivisible components called atoms.

Atrophy: partial or complete wasting away of parts of the body, e.g., muscles, from disuse.

Autonomic nervous system: part of the nervous system of the body which controls the 'fight or flight' response (sympathetic) as well as the 'rest and digest' or 'feed and breed' response (parasympathetic); previously thought to be beyond voluntary control.

B.C.E.: Before Common Era, formerly called 'BC'.

Biomedical: current dominating model of healthcare that defines health purely as an absence of illness.

Breech presentation: a baby positioned feet or bottom first in the uterus. A caesarean section is usually recommended for safe delivery.

Broad-spectrum: referring to antibiotics which target many commonly occurring infective agents. Overuse can cause imbalance in the gut flora and promote the development of drug resistant bacteria.

Bruxism: excessive teeth grinding or jaw clenching.

Bulimia: eating disorder characterised by binge eating followed by purging or fasting, related to excessive concern with body weight and shape.

Candidiasis: fungal infection caused by a yeast (Candida) affecting the mouth (thrush) or vagina; may spread to other parts of the body if the immune system is compromised.

Cardiovascular: relating to the heart and blood vessels.

Carbamate: pesticide similar to organophosphates used in agriculture which is toxic to humans.

Carnitine: a compound which supports energy production in skeletal and cardiac muscles.

CE: Common Era, formerly called 'AD'.

Chaste tree: botanical name *Vitex agnus-castus*; used in traditional herbal medicine for menstrual cycle hormonal regulation.

Cortex: the grey matter in the brain controlling memory, thinking, learning, reasoning, problem-solving, emotions and consciousness.

Cortisol: a steroid hormone produced in the adrenal gland, released in response to stress and low blood sugar levels; in excess can weaken the immune response.

Cytokines: a group of signalling proteins that help control inflammation in the body; in excess can cause auto-immune diseases.

Diaphragm: the dome-shaped muscle separating the chest and abdominal cavities.

Eleatic: pre-Socratic Greek philosophical school advocating a strict metaphysical view postulating a universal unity or divine influence separate from observed nature.

Electrolyte: mineral substance that has a natural positive or negative charge when dissolved in water, affecting the regulation of water content in the body and acidity of the blood.

Endocrine system: comprises the pituitary, pineal, thyroid, parathyroid, and adrenal glands as well as the ovaries and testes. They secrete hormones which target distant organs to regulate body functions.

Endorphins: a group of hormones which activate the body's opiate receptors causing an analgesic effect and an improved sense of wellbeing.

Eustress: meaning 'beneficial stress' – associated with release of feel-good chemicals like endorphins.

Fibromyalgia: muscle and fibrous connective tissue pain. A chronic medical condition characterised by widespread pain, fatigue, and sleep problems, believed to involve a combination of genetic and environmental factors (psychological stress, trauma, and certain infections).

Glycogen: stored glucose in the body found mainly in the liver and muscles.

Glucose: a simple sugar found in carbohydrates which is an important source of energy for the body.

Glutathione: an antioxidant.

Hippocratic medicine: a holistic health care model proposed by ancient Greek physician Hippocrates which emphasised professional integrity, benevolence, and human dignity in the practice of medicine, focused on understanding the consideration of the whole of a patient's health status.

Histamine: a compound produced by mast cells which mediates the allergic response.

Holistic medicine: a healthcare practice that considers the whole person – body, emotions, mind, and spirit – in the quest for optimal health and wellness.

Homeostasis: a condition of optimal functioning of the body reflected by maintaining variables like body temperature and fluid balance within certain pre-set limits.

Hylozoists: early Greek philosophical doctrine according to which all matter is alive.

Hyperarousal: a state of excessive psychological and physiological arousal (red alert) which can interfere with day-to-day life and sleep.

Hypertension: occurs when pressure in the blood vessels is too high, usually more than 140/90 or higher.

Hypoglycaemia: low blood sugar level; experienced as weakness, headaches, dizziness, blurred vision, confusion, and even fainting when severe.

Hypothalamus: almond-sized gland which links the nervous system to the endocrine system via the pituitary gland; it also regulates the functions of the autonomic nervous system.

Indole-3-carbinol: found in cruciferous vegetables (e.g., broccoli, cauliflower, and kale); used as a supplement to regulate oestrogen metabolism during the menstrual cycle and at menopause.

Inflammation: part of the complex biological response of body tissues to harmful stimuli, e.g., infection, which aims to eliminate the damage or injury caused by the initial triggering incident; signs are redness, pain, heat, swelling and loss of function.

Insulin: hormone produced by the pancreas which regulates metabolism of carbohydrates by promoting the absorption of glucose from the blood into the liver and muscles for storage as glycogen.

Integrative medicine: the medical practice of combining 'conventional' allopathic medicine with evidence-based complementary therapies to treat the whole person.

Isometric exercises: the repetitive tightening of a specific muscle or group of muscles which can help with maintaining or building strength.

Isonomia: the ancient Greek concept that equality of the opposing influences (wet-dry, cold-hot, bitter-sweet etc.) maintains health, while an imbalance of these causes illness.

Logos (Unity): ancient Greek concept of a universal divine reason, immanent in nature, yet transcending all opposites in the cosmos and humanity.

Lordosis: the inward curvature of the lumbar and cervical spines which when exaggerated by excess weight can result in muscle pain or spasm.

Mast cells: allergy cells responsible for immediate allergic reactions when they release chemicals like histamine in response to an allergen.

Meniscus: cartilage tissue that provides structural integrity to a joint during movement; a term usually used in reference to the knee joint.

Metabolism: chemical processes that occur in each cell, providing the body with life-giving energy.

Microbiome/Microflora: the trillions of micro-organisms of thousands of different species (bacteria, fungi, viruses, parasites) which live inside and on the body, the largest number being found in the gut. An imbalance between the helpful and the harmful types can lead to disease.

Micronutrient: substance required in trace amounts for normal growth and development, e.g., minerals and vitamins.

Milesian school: a philosophical school of ancient Greece that saw the world as a cosmos, an ordered arrangement that could be understood through rational inquiry.

Mitochondria: an organelle ('mini-organ') found in cells which generates chemical energy for growth and movement of the body.

Monosodium glutamate (MSG): a flavour enhancer often added to restaurant foods which can cause adverse reactions in sensitive individuals.

Morbidity: a state of being unhealthy from a disease.

Morton's neuroma: thickened fibrous tissue formed around a plantar nerve (in the foot) that results from compression between the toes from tight toe-box footwear and high heels; presents as pain and/or numbness in the affected toes.

Neuropeptides/Neurotransmitters: chemical messengers produced and co-released by nerve cells, acting as signalling molecules in the nervous system.

Nitric oxide: a signalling molecule which has effects on the nervous, immune, and cardiovascular systems. It dilates blood vessels, increasing blood flow.

Nocebo: opposite of placebo; any negative psychological or psychosomatic factor that produces a detrimental effect on health.

Nutraceutical: any product derived from food sources that brings health benefits in addition to its nutritional value.

Nystatin: antifungal medication used to treat Candida (yeast) infections.

Oncologist: a specialist doctor who treats cancer patients.

Organophosphates: organic pesticides used in agriculture, toxic to humans.

Osteoporosis: a medical condition of low bone density which in the elderly places them at risk of fractures.

Oxalic acid: implicated in formation of kidney stones; found in parsley, spinach, cassava, cabbage, broccoli, brussels sprouts, and quinoa.

Oxytocin: hormone produced in the deep brain (hypothalamus) that is involved in maternal bonding and milk production; also stimulates uterine contractions during childbirth.

Peroxynitrite: compound involved in reactions promoting cell damage.

Phenylalanine: an essential amino acid used as a supplement for its analgesic and anti-depressant effects.

Pituitary gland: endocrine gland located at the base of the brain secreting hormones which regulate important physiological processes e.g., stress, growth, reproduction, metabolism, and lactation.

Placebo: a medicine or procedure prescribed for psychological benefit rather than for any physiological effect.

Prebiotic: non-digestible components in foods that foster the growth or activity of beneficial bugs in the gut e.g., fermentable and starchy foods.

Probiotic: living micro-organisms beneficial to health found in foods such as yoghurt or available as supplements; recommended to restore balance in the gut after a course of broad-spectrum antibiotics.

Psychosomatic: relating to the interaction of mind (psyche) and body (somatic) on a physical illness.

Refined carbohydrates: sugars (e.g., sucrose, high-fructose corn syrup) and refined grains which have had the fibre and nutritional parts removed by processing, such as white bread, white rice, pastries, soda drinks, sweets, and some breakfast cereals. They are easily digested, causing rapid spikes in blood sugar levels.

Rhabdomyolysis: rapid breakdown of muscle tissues which can lead to kidney failure. Statin medication has been implicated as a cause in sensitive individuals.

Salicylates: chemicals found in fruits and vegetables, spices, herbs, and flavour additives. In sensitive individuals they can cause asthma flare-ups, skin rashes, headaches, gut disturbance, and behaviour problems in children.

Serotonin: a neurotransmitter modulating mood, learning, sleep, and memory functions.

Sodium benzoate: a food preservative (E211) found in salad dressings, carbonated soft drinks, jams, fruit juices, and pickles.

Sodium metabisulphite: another food and beverage (wine) preservative, with potential to harm some organs.

Tartrazine: a food colouring agent (E102) used mainly for yellow, found in desserts and confectionery, beverages, snacks, and condiments.

Temporomandibular joint: the joint between the jawbone (mandible) and the skull (temporal bone).

Theta brain waves: produced during dream-sleep and when awake but deeply relaxed.

Theobromine: an alkaloid compound obtained from cacao seeds, resembling caffeine in its effects.

Thymus gland: located in the upper front part of the chest behind the sternum, this gland supports the immune function up to the early teens when it starts to shrink.

Tyramine: an amino acid occurring naturally in the body but also found in aged cheese, cured or processed meats, pickled or fermented vegetables, and alcoholic beverages; can be a trigger for migraine headaches, and raises blood pressure.

Vasodilation: widening of blood vessels leading to increased blood flow.

Yin Yang: a concept in Chinese philosophy describing opposite but interconnected and mutually perpetuating forces. Yin is 'receptive' while Yang is 'active'.

INDEX

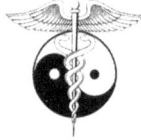

ABOUT THE AUTHOR

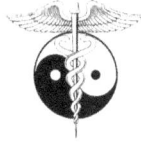

Dr Hira Singh (MBBS FRACGP) was born in Singapore where he completed his medical studies before migrating to Australia in 1977. He worked as a Country General Practitioner for ten years before establishing his Wholistic Medicine Clinic, combining Allopathic medicine with Acupuncture, Biofeedback, Stress Management (Meditation) Nutritional Medicine, Spinal Manipulation, and Counselling. With his integrative approach he has helped many to explore healing – which he defines as the optimal attunement of body, emotions, mind, and spirit.

He has lectured widely and presented his Whole Person Model of Care at conferences, both nationally and internationally.

He served as the Western Australian Representative on the Founding Board of the Australasian Integrative Medicine Association and as President of the Whole Health Institute.

NOTES

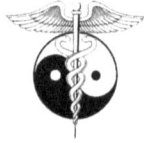

NOTES

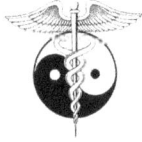